ALZH[...]

THE COMPL[...]
FOR FAMILIES
AND LOVED ONES

Updated and Revised

Howard Gruetzner, M.Ed.

Director, Elder Services
Heart of Texas Region MHMR Center

John Wiley & Sons, Inc.
New York • Chichester • Weinheim • Brisbane • Singapore • Toronto

To Bob Herbert,
a dedicated warrior for the welfare
of the community and its people

This publication is provided to serve the reader as a supplement to professional medical guidance and treatment, and not as a substitute for professional medical care. As new medical research broadens our knowledge, changes in treatment and drug therapy are required. The author and publisher have made every effort to ensure that information regarding medical treatment is accurate and in accordance with the standards accepted at the time of publication. Readers are advised, however, to follow the product information sheet included with any drug administered and to seek professional advice before proceeding with medical treatment.

This book was sponsored by
  Heart of Texas Region Mental Health Mental Retardation Center, Waco, Texas
                      and
  DePaul Center (A division of Providence Hospital, Daughters of Charity of St. Vincent DePaul), Waco, Texas

Library of Congress Cataloging-in-Publication Data:
Gruetzner, Howard.
      Alzheimer's: the complete guide for family and loved ones / Howard Gruetzner. — updated and revised
          p.   cm.
      Includes bibliographical references (p.   ) and index
      ISBN 0-471-56884-8 (pbk.)
      ISBN 0-471-19825-0 (mass market)
  1. Alzheimer's disease. I. Title
RC523.G78   1992
362.1'96831-dc20   92-3807

Printed in the United States of America

10 9 8 7 6 5 4 3 2 1

CONTENTS

PREFACE

In the United States today, there are more than two million victims of Alzheimer's disease, and the number is growing. The disease eventually renders the brain virtually useless, and it turns lives inside out—both the lives of the people who have Alzheimer's and the lives of those closest to them. It is a slow, as yet irreversible, disease that ulitmately leads to death.

However, families confronted with Alzheimer's disease no longer must struggle through this difficult illness alone. Tremendous advances have been made in recent years in understanding the disease and devising successful care and management techniques—information that is presented in readily and understandable terms in *ALZHEIMER'S: A Caregiver's Guide and Sourcebook*. With this book as a companion, caring for an Alzheimer's patient can be a far more positive experience than families could have thought possible.

This book can give both families and professionals a better understanding of the disease, of the victim's behavior, and of ways to cope effectively with the demands of caring for Alzheimer's patients. The first ten chapters, based primarily on the author's fifteen years of specialized work with the elderly mentally-ill population in Central Texas, cover symptoms and stages of Alzheimer's and provide an overview of what to expect as the illness progresses. A special section explores the full range of resources for Alzheimer's care available in a community—resources that can provide families with much-appreciated relief from the burdens of daily care. The book also includes tips on locating resources such as diagnosis, home health services, and nursing home placements, as well as helpful suggestions on reducing caregiver stress.

Possible causes of Alzheimer's disease are considered in Part I. This discussion also addresses psychosocial factors that relate to this illness. Research is beginning to make some progress that broadens our knowledge of Alzheimer's disease. Other aspects of research are considered in Part II. Two chapters are designed to acquaint both caregivers and professionals with what actually happens in the brain as Alzheimer's disease progresses. Overviews of current drug treatment research, as well as other research findings that may contribute to treatment, are included.

Care management of the dementia patient can often benefit from careful use of traditional psychiatric medications. These medications, by providing helpful ways to reduce behavioral and emotional manifestations of the disease, may also extend the period of time the affected individual can be cared for in the home appropriately. With an understanding of care management principles outlined in this book and active utilization of existing resources, caregivers will be better equipped to cope with the physical and emotional challenge confronting them. Psychiatric medications are best used in this broader context of caregiving.

This updated and revised edition includes three new chapters: Chapters 7, 9, and 12. Chapter 7 discusses how behavioral changes associated with Alzheimer's disease challenge family caregivers, who must rethink their assumptions about behaviors and what causes them. The victim's behavior is eventually a function of external factors, and views about "self-control" must be revised.

Chapter 9 considers how families are affected by the Alzheimer's situation. Different types of families approach the Alzheimer's crisis in different ways. Different roles are assumed by family members, and these roles are not always supportive of caregiving. The chapter also examines the balancing of caring with caregiving.

Behavioral changes also suggest that the person is no longer who he or she used to be. This recognition triggers the grief process that is so much a part of Alzheimer's caregiving. Chapter 12, "Getting Help" examines the role of grief in caregiver's help-seeking efforts.

It is hoped that this guide will serve as a comprehensive reference that will make the caregiver's tasks easier, more rewarding, and more constructive. In turn, we hope it will help to make the lives of those caught in the grip of Alzheimer's disease happier, safer, and more comfortable.

ACKNOWLEDGMENTS

I am especially grateful to family, personal friends, and professional colleagues who gave their support to this book. Observing the challenges of caring for a relative with dementia has been both revealing and rewarding. Much more information than ever before is available now for families caring for loved ones who have Alzheimer's disease. When I began to work with people who had dementia in the early 1970s, the attitudes toward dementia were reflective of the negative social attitudes we had toward our aging citizens. It was not a comprehensive, sensitive approach to evaluation and treatment.

I am indebted to the staff of a local psychiatric hospital, De Paul Center, a division of Providence Hospital, Daughters of Charity of St. Vincent de Paul, and the psychiatrists associated with that hospital who provided helpful comments on the manuscript. The psychiatrists who took time to read the manuscript and comment include: Stephen Mark, M.D.; Bergen Morrison, M.D.; Thomas Stidvent, M.D.; and Jack Wentworth, M.D. I also appreciate other encouraging comments from Rod Ryan, M.D., family practice physician.

Dennis Myers, Ph.D., of the Baylor University Institute of Gerontological Studies used the section dealing with matters relevant to caregiving in a mental health and aging course. I appreciate Dr. Myer's comments and those of his students regarding the book's usefulness as a text. Martie Sauter of the McLennan Community College Mental Health Associates Degree Program was very generous in describing the book's usefulness for training students and caregivers.

To make the chapters dealing with scientific studies on research and treatment comprehensible and meaningful required considerable simplification. One risk of simplifying such material is that its accuracy may be compromised. I appreciate the comments made by a number of physicians including a neurosurgeon, R. H. Saxton, M.D.;

a neurologist, Mark Schwartze, M.D.; a family practice physician, Edward Cooney, M.D.; a radiologist, R. L. Zeigler, M.D. The comments of Charles Conley, M.D., a pathologist, were extremely helpful. Bill Kersh, a biologist, reviewed sections concerning the chemical changes in the brain.

Hazel Limback, Deputy Executive Director of Heart of Texas Council of Governments, Area Agency of Aging, gave consistent support and encouragement to this project. I appreciate her concern for persons affected by Alzheimer's disease and their needs. I also appreciate the interest shown by planners from the State of Texas, Office of the Governor and Texas Department of Aging concerning the special needs created by this disease.

Danny Fred provided tireless assistance with typing, rewriting, and editing. One of my colleagues, Samantha Anderson, provided helpful assistance with the editing and rewriting. Jeanne Levy spent extra hours typing the first draft of the section on research and treatment, which no doubt seemed to have been written in a foreign language. I appreciate other typing assistance from a friend, Pam Richard, R.N., who unselfishly provided her time and support.

Katherine Gregor edited the final manuscript with professional objectivity, clarity, and sensitivity. Lynn Pearson provided tireless assistance with typing, rewriting, and editing for the entire book. She was especially helpful in keeping the manuscript simple and readable.

Staff of MHMR Aging Services provided more support than they know in attending to the needs of our clients. I appreciate Vanessa Hummel, Terry Brandon, Melissa Talamantes, and Melba Ogle.

Much of the research for this and the first edition was conducted at the library of the Veteran's Administration Medical Center in Waco, Texas. I am in the debt of the library staff of that facility, especially to Barbara Hobbs. I am also grateful to Ginger Kirkland, R.N., for her timely research assistance and her continual support. A longtime friend, Vicki Cotrell, Ph.D., was helpful in formulating some of the more difficult concepts important to include in this edition.

When one is putting together ideas for a project like this, family and friends must be willing to accept the "enforced" isolation this entails. I appreciate the many gestures of support from these individuals. Patty Hawk's editing of new chapters was sensitive and supportive of the ideas I wanted to convey. Ted Scheffler, my editor at Wiley, gave encouragement and support for the new chapters. As before, I am grateful to Nancy Marcus Land with Publications

Development Company of Texas, for her assistance in the production of this book.

I want to thank my many clients and their families. They have entrusted their problems and needs to strangers, and as someone who must begin professional relationships as a stranger, I appreciate what can be learned from these other "strangers," our clients and families.

As a Director of a Geriatric Mental Health Program, I can't fool myself. When all is said and done, the knowledge that clients and their families received quality care and services makes an important difference. My thanks goes to our staff: Nata Boone, Curtis Garner, Sandra Priest, Angie Scott, Angela Antis, David Beyer, M.D., and Swamji Badhiwala, M.D.

I am very pleased that Wiley has made it possible for this book to be read by more people encountering Alzheimer's. I want to thank Tom Miller, my Senior Editor, for his support and assistance in revisions to the text that update the reader on what is new. Finally, I thank my wife, Ginger, for her support of me, the writing, and the reasons that are important to me.

SPECIAL ACKNOWLEDGMENT

About the Poetry

MAUDE NEWTON has survived one of the most difficult experiences life can hand a person: watching her husband, Frank, move slowly, progressively toward death. Frank Newton, who had retired from a successful career in banking, real estate, and insurance in Del Rio, TX, had Alzheimer's disease.

As Mrs. Newton went through all of the disease's stages with her husband, she began an intimate chronicle of her thoughts and feelings in verse form.

"I started picking up whatever was handy—the backs of envelopes, notepaper, whatever—to write about how I was feeling at that moment," she said. "I found it was doing me a lot of good. I was verbalizing my feelings, even if just on a piece of paper." Her children insisted she save all her scibbled thoughts: later, they typed, copied, and bound the collection. Mrs. Newton's poetry introduces a number of issues in a personal, moving way, and we thank her for allowing us to reprint a few of her poems.

PART I

THE CAREGIVER EXPERIENCE

Alzheimer's disease cannot be cured. Part I focuses on what we know about this disease and what we can do to care for individuals thought to have Alzheimer's. A better understanding of this condition and its behavioral manifestations enables caregivers to respond more effectively to the needs of loved ones.

Our beliefs about the Alzheimer's patient and his behavior do not take into account the effects of brain impairment. We have no frame of reference through which brain-impaired behavior can be understood. Part I provides this perspective so that caregivers can more effectively and positively respond to the problems and needs of their loved ones.

The caregiver experience is characterized by the adjustment of the Alzheimer's patient and his family to this illness. Part I will examine this adjustment in several ways. Stages of the illness and the family adjustment will be considered. A step-by-step guide describes the experience from the time initial symptoms are noticed to the point care is planned and caregiver stress encountered. Practical approaches to these steps are considered. Community resources are described in the last chapter of Part I since social support is such an important way for caregivers to provide for the increasing needs of their loved ones and themselves.

TWILIGHT

It's that time again,
that time when day fades into night . . .
that time when—
if you were working late
(and I had a few minutes to wait),
I'd pick up the papers on the floor,
fluff up the pillows a bit,
and open the door to look for you.
It was good to sit on the sofa
and feel you close—
to hear about your day
and share mine with you.

It was always my favorite time of the day
when the bustle gave way
to the shared things we used to say.

Now I dread it—
I hate to sit and watch it come on—
without you.
It's just a time I must learn to endure—
to live through.

Maude S. Newton

1

WHAT IS ALZHEIMER'S DISEASE?

A case history Jewell Johnson had once been quite active in her neighborhood. She had also attended church regularly. These activities had not significantly changed following her husband's death three years earlier. Her friends and family had been impressed with how well she made it through the grief and kept her life going. She had always been stronger and healthier than her husband. Mrs. Johnson was now 74 and seemed to be a model for aging.

Uncharacteristic behavior is noticed. Several months ago her closest neighbors began to notice changes. First, she dropped out of church. They discovered that her feelings had been hurt. Apparently, she had made some mistakes as the treasurer of her Sunday School class, losing several hundred dollars. That was not her story, though; Mrs. Johnson insisted that someone had stolen the money. It had all been cash, and for some reason she had never deposited it in the bank.

She began to stay home more and more often. It also surprised the neighbors that she discouraged their visits. They were becoming worried about her and considered calling relatives, but her son and daughter both lived several hundred miles away and telephoned regularly. Their professional jobs made it difficult to visit very often. The pastor tried to visit, but Jewell was uncharacteristically rude to him and other church members who tried to visit her.

Household chores and personal hygiene are neglected.

The yard was still covered with leaves left since the fall. It was now the middle of winter. On occasion, neighbors would check on Jewell. Several times a week her morning newspapers remained in the yard, and this gave neighbors an excuse to check on her. She always came to the door in her robe and slippers. She thanked them for the paper, making excuses that she had a cold and was resting more. She refused their offers to help her. If they pursued these offers too long, she would become more restless and agitated. A few times she had shut the door abruptly.

Her closest next-door neighbor called the daughter, Joan. Joan was caught off guard because the phone conversations with her mother—while briefer and more vague—had not been that different. Her mother had always been self-reliant and independent; it was no surprise that she was so reluctant to accept help. It was strange that Jewell never told her daughter of any problems. Maybe that was why the conversations were briefer and so general. The neighbor was asked to watch after Jewell, and the daughter called her mother.

Behavior changes are denied.

This was not a pleasant conversation, nor was it very long. Jewell denied any problems and told her daughter the neighbor was meddling. Jewell thought the neighbor's son was trying to get her house. The next-door neighbor had never been honest. As the paranoia became more vivid, Jewell became more upset and hung up on the daughter. Joan called the neighbor and said she would be down the following weekend.

Bills remain unpaid.

The next day both the gas and electric company cut off their services to Jewell's home. In the dead of winter, they do not usually cut off the services of elderly people. The neighbor argued on Jewell's behalf but to no avail. She had not paid her bills for more than three months (about the same time she stopped attending church). Attempts to get Mrs. Johnson to the door failed. She would look out the window briefly, but that was all she would do. No one could get into the house. Neighbors called the daughter, but they could think of nothing else that would help.

Delusions develop.

Late that night, the neighbors were awakened by screaming outside Jewell's house. It was nearly freezing, and she was outside her home in a gown. She was afraid of the neighbors who tried to help calm her. She kept talking about her husband roaming around in the attic. She was afraid of him. The police were called and when they arrived on the scene, Mrs. Johnson was frightened and still very upset. She was quite confused and could only talk about her husband in the attic. They investigated and found no sign of anyone in the attic—just as they had expected. A crisis hot line was called, and Mrs. Johnson was hospitalized since she had become a danger to herself.

Closer examination of the household was revealing. There was not any food in the household. She probably had not eaten anything to speak of for several days. The kitchen was a mess, and the gas burners were still turned on although gas service had been terminated. The police explored the rest of the household. Clothes were lying around. The toilet had not been flushed for days, and Mrs. Johnson had had some accidents in her bedroom. Newspapers lay on the living room floor rolled up and unread. Bills and other mail were heaped in piles near the newspapers.

After being stabilized in the psychiatric hospital, a thorough examination was conducted. Upon its completion, only one conclusion could explain what had happened to Mrs. Jewell Johnson over the past year to six months. Something had obviously been happening before her behavior changes suggested something was wrong. In fact, it was admirable that she had so successfully compensated for the difficulties she was experiencing in memory and thinking. The diagnosis was inescapable—probable Alzheimer's disease.

It was 1980, and her family and friends were bewildered. They had never heard of Alzheimer's disease. They had been prepared to accept a diagnosis of "senility." Maybe her problems could be explained by depression or old age. The friends of Jewell Johnson and her family began to try to understand what was happening and what would be done.

Alzheimer's disease? That sounds so strange and terrible. What is Alzheimer's disease?

Alzheimer's disease is a condition of unknown origin that causes gradual loss of abilities in memory, thinking, reasoning, judgment, orientation, and concentration. Alzheimer's disease is not the result of normal aging, but it does occur more frequently in persons who are 65 years of age or older.

More than simple forgetfulness

Alzheimer's disease is far more serious than the occasional forgetfulness experienced by the elderly. In its early stages, however, the disease can be difficult to distinguish from ordinary forgetfulness. The disease affects the brain gradually, and persons ordinarily will compensate for the early symptoms; thus neither the victim nor those around her may suspect a medical problem at first. The results of Alzheimer's slow but progressive damage to the brain often are not noticed until the person experiences greater than normal stress, pressures, or losses that stretch her coping abilities to the breaking point, or until the damage to the brain reaches an advanced stage.

Causes of disease unknown

Although much is known about the symptoms of the disease, little is known of the causes. Ongoing research is being conducted toward unlocking the secret of the disease, but at present neither a full scientific understanding nor a cure exists.

Research has revealed differences in the brains of persons with this disease such as abnormal proteins and higher concentrations of aluminum. Nonetheless, it is not known whether these abnormalities are a cause or result of the disease process. Since there is no cure, treatment consists of symptom management and overall care of the person.

The disease was first identified in 1906 by a German neurologist, Alois Alzheimer (pronounced Altz-hi-merz). His subject was a 51-year-old woman who exhibited problems with memory and disorientation. Later, Alzheimer identified depression and hallucinations as additional symptoms. The woman's condition continued to deteriorate; a severe dementia was evident, and the woman eventually died. An autopsy of the woman revealed that her brain had cortical atrophy and abnormalities in the cerebral cortex called neurofibrillary tangles. These changes in the brain were thought to have caused the impairment of the woman's memory, her disorientation, and her cognitive and emotional decline.

Causes of the symptoms in older people attributed to other causes

Because Alzheimer's disease was originally identified in persons under 60 and other causes were considered for similar symptoms in older persons, it was thought to be rare. It wasn't until the 1970's that several investigations led to the conclusion that Alzheimer's disease was accountable for the symptoms found in older persons (Katzman 1976).

Four million people in the United States affected

Twenty-five million Americans are now 65 years of age and older and it is estimated that 4 million Americans have Alzheimer's Disease (Weiner 1996). The incidence of the disease for persons who are 65 and older is nearly 10 percent. The incidence increases with age. For example, from 20 to 47 percent of persons over age 85 have dementia; of this number, Alzheimer's disease accounts for over 50 percent. By the year 2000 as many as five million cases of Alzheimer's disease can be anticipated (Weiner 1996). Alzheimer's disease is the most common neurological disease that causes dementia, a brain condition that results in a loss of intellectual capacities and impairs both social and occupational functioning. The incidence of the disease in women is a little higher than in men. The disease knows no socioeconomic boundaries. Once a person develops Alzheimer's, his or her life expectancy is reduced by approximately one-third. The average duration of the illness is from 4 to 8 years. The rate of deterioration and the severity vary with the individual. Some people have had the disease for as long as twenty years.

Cost of Alzheimer's disease

Alzheimer's disease is the fourth leading cause of death in the United States, killing more than 100,000 people annually. Doctors and coroners use different criteria for diagnosing dementia and attribute the cause of death to other causes, like respiratory conditions and infections, which often develop in the late stages of the disease. More than 50 percent of persons in nursing homes are afflicted with Alzheimer's. Alzheimer's care is estimated to cost America nearly $100 billion a year (Weiner 1996). The cost experienced by the individuals directly affected by Alzheimer's goes deeper: loss of self and long good-byes.

WHY?

I've heard it said,
"If there weren't a God
we would invent one,
for in our hour of deepest need
we must have someone—
some power on which to call."

I don't know . . .
I try hard to believe—
but we are rational creatures.
I must think,
or why was I given a mind?

I think and think
and it makes no sense.
Why would a loving Father
do this to my mate?
Why would he take from him
his mind—his pride
in being alive?

Why would he rob from him
his joy in being here?
Why leave him thus—
a poor shambling caricature
of the man he was?

Surely not for my sake—
to test my power to believe.
If so, it has defeated its purpose.
It's left me tormented and vulnerable
seeking an answer—and finding none—
and calling out—
"Oh, God—if you are my God, Why?"

Maude S. Newton

2

SYMPTOMS AND PHASES OF ALZHEIMER'S DISEASE

Symptoms of Alzheimer's Disease

Alzheimer's disease: a neurological condition causing deficient thinking and remembering

Alzheimer's disease is a neurological condition that impairs the brain's functioning. (Its exact cause is not known, but the leading theories will be explored in Chapter 4 and 14.) Symptoms of the illness represent deficits in many areas of how a person remembers and thinks. For instance, problems with memory may be manifested as forgetting names, dates, places, whether a bill has been paid, or something said over and over. Intellectual abilities are lost eventually. Reasoning with the affected person is no longer a successful way to understand and deal with his problems. Judgment about common everyday situations is drastically diminished. The individual's capacity to express himself verbally gradually shrinks. Neither is he able to comprehend what others say to him. As the disease progresses, he may gradually lose the ability to speak. Psychiatric symptoms such as delusions and hallucinations can occur. The person can become anxious, restless, agitated, and may even appear to be depressed. His personality will change. In fact, he may not seem to be the same person. What kind of disease is Alzheimer's disease?

Alzheimer's disease produces symptoms that are characteristic of a syndrome known as *dementia*. This type of condition was inaccurately labeled in the past as senility by both professionals and the public when older persons became forgetful and were unable to adequately care for themselves. Several labels may still be applied to

9

cases of Alzheimer's disease. Organic brain syndrome, senile dementia, and degenerative dementia have been used in the past. The preferred diagnostic term is now *dementia of the Alzheimer's type*.

Dementia: loss of intellectual abilities

Dementia, in its broader sense, indicates a loss or impairment of a person's abilities to use his mind. The essential feature of dementia is a loss of intellectual abilities severe enough to interfere with social or occupational functioning. An accountant with Alzheimer's disease will be unable to perform his job because of impairments in memory, reasoning, and calculation abilities. A farmer will become unable to plant and harvest crops. Buying seed and figuring out how much seed to put in planters or drills will become impossible.

Alzheimer's disease is the most common type of dementia. It is not, however, the only dementing illness. Multiple strokes can create a dementia that resembles Alzheimer's disease. Depression and other psychiatric conditions can produce conditions that look like dementia. In the elderly, severe depresson is a psychiatric condition that looks like dementia. This condition used to be called a pseudodementia or "false" dementia. It had symptoms like dementia but could usually be treated successfully. Underlying medical conditions can cause some symptoms that suggest dementia—for example, vitamin B-12 deficiencies, thyroid disturbances, and pernicious anemia. Proper treatment usually reverses the symptoms that resemble dementia. When symptoms do not respond to treatment as expected, the suspicion that Alzheimer's is present increases.

Other causes of the dementia must first be ruled out.

At this time there is no definitive medical test that can diagnose Alzheimer's disease. Other potential causes of dementia must be ruled out. This is extremely important, not only to arrive at a correct diagnosis, but to identify any treatable condition. The coexistence of several conditions may cause dementia. Even if one condition, such as Alzheimer's disease, cannot be treated in the sense of cured or slowed, it is important to treat the conditions which can be managed. The treatment will very likely improve the individual's functioning to some degree, despite the fact that he has a progressive dementing illness. Alzheimer's disease is a probable diagnosis given only after all other potential causes of dementia have been identified and treated or ruled out. This is one major reason the diagnostic process is a collaborative effort.

The diagnostic criteria for dementia of the Alzheimer's type as specified by DSM–IV (American Psychiatric Association 1994) stipulate symptoms and how they can be recognized and measured by a person involved in the diagnostic process. Multiple cognitive deficits must have developed and be manifested by both (1) memory impairment and (2) one or more of the following cognitive disturbances: aphasia, apraxia, agnosia, and/or a disturbance in executive functioning. Executive functioning is defined as cognitive abilities that involve planning, organizing, sequencing, and abstracting. Other conditions must also be met. For instance, the course of the disease must be characterized by a gradual onset and continuing cognitive decline, and not be due to other known medical or psychiatric conditions.

First criteria for dementia: severe loss of intellectual functioning

The first criteria for dementia is the *loss of intellectual abilities* of sufficient severity to interfere with social or occupational functioning. This indicates that not only are these abilities impaired, but they also must be affected to the degree that the person cannot perform usual work-related activities satisfactorily. For instance, a teacher will be unable to prepare lessons and keep his presentations to the class organized and comprehensible. He may be unable to provide information that was very easy for him to grasp before the Alzheimer's process began. New academic demands may become quite stressful. In social situations he may have trouble following conversations and become confused by new points of discussion. Social demands can become more troublesome, and he may withdraw or become more anxious in social situations. His responses to other people may make less sense and not be very well related to a topic of conversation.

Routine activities become increasingly difficult.

As Alzheimer's disease progresses, a person's ability to successfully carry out familiar activities of daily living will decline. The thinking abilities required to cook a meal, pay bills, clean house, bathe, dress, or even dial a telephone will diminish gradually. Because of memory problems, the person may also claim that tasks have been done, although it is quite evident they have not.

Severe memory problems are often the earliest symptoms.

Memory impairment has many manifestations during the course of Alzheimer's disease. Forgetfulness is often listed as a condition of old age, and in fact some memory loss is normal in later years. Misplacing keys or a checkbook is something all of us have experienced, regardless of our age. The memory impairment that occurs with Alzheimer's disease is much more pervasive and disabling. Problems with memory are usually the earliest and most obvious symptom of this condition. It is also a symptom that is often denied by individuals with Alzheimer's disease.

Ability to remember recently received information is affected first.

Recent memory, that is, memory for events and information experienced over the past half hour, is most affected earlier in Alzheimer's. Such memory loss obviously affects a person's daily living circumstances. Bills are not paid, the gas may be left on, appointments are missed, or keeping track of a daily routine is disturbed. Immediate recall is the ability to repeat something that has just been said. Persons with Alzheimer's disease may have good immediate recall, but little information is likely to be remembered later. New information is not easily remembered.

New learning affected

Recent memory problems also make it difficult for persons with an Alzheimer's-type dementia to learn new material or activities. For example, keeping up with time and place, learning new names, or remembering a shopping list, which involve recent memory abilities, become increasingly difficult as the disease progresses. Disorientation, which involves forgetting time, person, and place, can occur in Alzheimer's disease. For example, the person will reach a point when he cannot remember the day of the week, the month, or the year. Such disorientation and memory problems will contribute to the person's getting lost and will be especially evident in new situations or places.

Memories of past remain longer.
Remote memory is the person's grasp of his past. For instance, this involves information about where he was born, when he was born, his parents and siblings, where he attended school, and when he graduated from school. Personal history is recorded in remote memory. Remote memory also includes facts about past presidents, wars, economic, and political events. In the early stages of Alzheimer's disease, remote memory is less obviously affected but becomes more noticeably impaired over time. Direct questions or confrontations will expose gaps that exist in remote memory. Distant memories may serve as a refuge when recent memory becomes so severely affected the individual cannot relate to what is currently happening.

Maintenance of daily routines is helpful for memory-impaired persons. Such routines can help organize a life that has become unpredictable and insecure because failing memory cannot assist the individual in controlling daily events and interactions.

The loss of intellectual functioning and impaired memory are essential ingredients in an Alzheimer's-type dementia, but several other symptoms of dementia must also be present. Some of these do not occur until later in the course of the illness and may vary considerably from one person to the next. At least one of the following symptoms must be present for primary degenerative dementia to be diagnosed.

Faulty judgment puts Alzheimer's patients in dangerous situations
Impaired judgment and insight are symptoms which are manifested in the lives of persons with Alzheimer's disease. Impaired judgment occurs in many areas of the person's life and can lead to dangerous consequences. For example, the person may insist on driving the car when it is clear his ability has been seriously impaired. He may insist he can manage his finances as well as anyone, even when obviously he cannot. Cooking and lighting stoves are activities where poor judgment may become evident as well as dangerous.

Of course, the dementing process is responsible for impaired judgment. However, some environments encourage rather than restrict the exercise of poor judgment. Some caregivers may be understandably anxious about confronting these kinds of behaviors, but the need to intervene usually increases with the potential risks to the Alzheimer's patient, especially when they carry with them risks to other persons. (Driving is a good example of this type of situation.)

Abilities to discern differences and similarities between things decrease.

Impairment of abstract thinking is more difficult to recognize in everyday actions. It is more easily assessed by answers to certain types of questions. For example, proverbs such as "Haste makes waste" are difficult for persons with dementia to adequately explain. The similarities and differences between things cannot be discerned. A chair and desk are alike because both are furniture. Such associations are not likely to be made by the person with Alzheimer's disease. Defining words and concepts are other examples of tasks that require abstract thinking or reasoning.

Alzheimer's disease affects the cortex of the brain. The cortex is discussed more specifically in Chapter 14, but we should make one point here. There are several human functions controlled by the cortex, the brain's outer layer. Some of these functions involve speech and movement abilities.

Aphasia, a problem with speaking and understanding language, develops.

One disturbance of cortical functioning associated with Alzheimer's disease is called *aphasia*. Aphasia is the loss of previously possessed abilities in language comprehension or production. Because of damage to the brain, an individual is unable to understand speech. Verbal expression also becomes disturbed in Alzheimer's disease. These speech deficits do not occur abruptly, as is common with a stroke. Speech abilities are gradually eroded. Individual variations occur during the disease process, but usually speech problems begin with some difficulty in word-finding. When talking, the person may have trouble making a point or answering a question directly. Spontaneous speech can be wordy and evasive. His comments wander around the point but never get to it. Later, word-finding problems and inability to name objects become very apparent.

Comprehension of what others say becomes impaired; thus the person is reluctant to engage in conversation. Spoken words or combinations of words are also misused. Later, even misused words have less meaningful relationships to the words for which they are substituted. The person may even echo what is said to him. Finally, the ability to produce sounds and words is reduced because the person is having difficulty coordinating his speech apparatus. The complete inability to speak will occur in many persons during the very last stage of Alzheimer's disease.

Difficulties in performing purposeful movement, apraxia, become evident.

Additionally, difficulties in movement can occur with Alzheimer's disease. One such impairment of movement is called *apraxia*. Apraxia is the loss of a previously possessed ability to perform skilled and purposeful motor acts. It is not the result of weakness but rather brain damage which prevents a person from making an intended movement. It is sometimes hard to determine whether Alzheimer's patients have trouble dressing themselves because of memory problems and the inability to grasp the logical sequence of the task or because they are exhibiting apraxia. Later in the illness, difficulties in grasping a fork, spoon, or cup, and carrying out intended movements could be due to apraxia.

Inability to recognize objects and people, agnosia, occurs.

Agnosia, an inability to recognize objects and people, is another brain disturbance in Alzheimer's disease. Agnosia is not a memory problem. Brain damage makes it impossible for information to be processed correctly. Visual information is distorted by the brain so that it is unrecognizable. The affected person may not recognize his home. At times, he may ask where his spouse is even though that spouse is sitting close by.

Number skills diminish and are lost.

The ability to do mathematic calculations is also lost with Alzheimer's disease. This is not merely a problem with memory; number skills are simply lost. Addition, subtraction, and other mathematical operations cannot be done successfully.

Such problems create obstacles to successful daily living, particularly in paying bills and keeping checking accounts balanced. If the person is employed in a job that requires the use of mathematics, calculation problems may emerge before other problems are evident. This includes sales clerks as well as accountants.

Writing skills progressively erode. Writing abilities will ultimately be impaired. Initially the person may have some trouble writing paragraphs which require him to keep up with a lot of information. Gradually the ability to write sentences will erode. Words may be used incorrectly and misspelled. Eventually the person will be unable to write his name. Reading abilities may be intact longer, although grasping the meaning of what has been read disappears sooner because of memory and intellectual problems.

Another symptom of an Alzheimer's-type dementia is difficulty in drawing and copying geometric designs. Three dimensional figures are especially difficult to reproduce. The ability to draw or copy simpler figures will deteriorate as the disease progresses. Loss of these abilities may not seem significant, but the general loss of visual-spatial skills does impact daily living. Writing, reading, finding one's way in a neighborhood, or locating items in the home all involve visual-spatial abilities.

Personality changes become noticeable early. *Personality changes* occur with dementia. Usually these changes become evident after the very early stages of the illness. Some personality changes may be a reaction to unsuccessful compensations for losses in functioning; brain damage also alters the personality. With Alzheimer's disease, personality traits may become more evident and actually be accentuated. A suspicious person will probably become frankly paranoid. An individual who has always reacted strongly to little troubles will react more often and more strongly to small problems. The individual's personality will change as a result of the progressive brain damage, and the person will not seem to be himself.

Before making a diagnosis of dementia, delirium must be ruled out.

One final condition, along with the confirmation of the previously described symptoms, must be met for a diagnosis of dementia to be possible. The individual must *show clear consciousness,* which means there is no evidence that delirium is creating the symptoms. Delirium is a clouding of one's consciousness, with a decreased awareness of his immediate environment. A person who is delirious finds it difficult to shift, focus, and sustain attention to what is occurring in his environment. His perceptions of these occurrences are disturbed. Speech may be incoherent. Disorientation and memory impairment may be present, but they are caused by the delirium, not by the dementia. Persons with Alzheimer's disease may suffer delirium at times because of underlying infections or other medical problems, which make the dementia appear to have worsened.

The symptoms we have discussed represent criteria for professionals to diagnose dementia. However, before a diagnosis can be made, the cause of the dementia must be determined. There are many conditions that can cause dementia. Alzheimer's disease may be more common, but it can only be given as a probable diagnosis when all other conditions are appropriately excluded. The history of the symptoms is extremely important since some dementing conditions such as strokes occur abruptly. In others, like Parkinson's disease, dementia develops over a period of time comparable to Alzheimer's disease. Even if other potential causes for dementia have been ruled out, one must monitor the course of the condition. In some cases the progression may move very rapidly or seem to stop. Such phenomena may require some cases to be reconsidered. Severe depression may mimic dementia, but, with treatment, the dementia-like symptoms may improve.

Dementia can be caused by treatable conditions.

Some conditions that cause dementia can be treated successfully, thus reversing the dementia. We will list some of the more common of these treatable conditions. The reader should note that the conditions listed do not inevitably cause dementia, and that some conditions also can cause delirium.

Reversible Causes of Dementia Symptoms and Delirium

	Delirium	Dementia
Depression		Yes
Congestive Heart Failure	Yes	Yes
Acute Myocardial Infarct	Yes	
Renal Failure	Yes	Yes
Hypoglycemia	Yes	Yes
Hyperglycemia	Yes	Yes
Hypothyroidism	Yes	Yes
Hyperthyroidism	Yes	Yes
Pneumonia	Yes	
Diverticulitis	Yes	
Transient Ischemia	Yes	
Stroke	Yes	Yes
Subdural Hematoma	Yes	Yes
Concussion	Yes	
Neurosyphilis	Yes	Yes
Tuberculosis	Yes	Yes
Brain Tumor	Yes	Yes
Brain Abscess	Yes	Yes
Normal Pressure Hydrocephalus (abnormal flow of spinal fluid)		Yes
Fecal Impaction	Yes	
Urinary Retention	Yes	
Sensory Deprivation States (such as blindness or deafness)	Yes	Yes
Environmental Changes and Isolation	Yes	Yes
Electrolyte Abnormalities		Yes
Lifelong Alcoholism		Yes
Anemia	Yes	Yes
Chronic Lung Disease with Hypoxia	Yes	Yes
Deficiencies of Nutrients (such as vitamins B-12, folic acid, niacin)		Yes
Drug intoxication	Yes	Yes
Bladder, Urinary Tract Infection	Yes	

This list of conditions, while incomplete, illustrates the fact that a number of conditions can cause both dementia and delirium. It would be tragic for a diagnosis of Alzheimer's disease or another irreversible dementia to be given without the proper physical examination, laboratory, and other diagnostic tests being completed. Such tests may reveal that a person has a treatable condition. The importance of the appropriate medical personnel being involved in some part of the evaluation of dementia cannot be stressed enough.

Along with these treatable conditions, other irreversible dementias (those that cannot be treated) must be considered. Alzheimer's disease is the most common irreversible dementia, followed by multi-infarct dementia, which is caused by multiple strokes. About 50 percent of all dementias of the elderly are caused by Alzheimer's disease; 20 percent to 25 percent are caused by multi-infarct disease, and another 20 percent of dementias are caused by a combination of these two conditions. Other conditions account for less than 10 percent of dementias. The following list illustrates some of these irreversible dementias. We will list only the more commonly known conditions. Of course, some of these are still quite rare, for example, Creutzfeldt-Jakob disease and Pick's disease. General Paresis, which is a form of central nervous system syphilis, is becoming rare with the successful treatment of syphilis.

Irreversible Dementias

Alzheimer's Disease
Pick's Disease
Vascular Dementia
Creutzfeldt-Jakob Disease
Kuru
General Paresis
Parkinson's Disease
Huntington's Disease
Wilson's Disease
Binswanger's Disease

Vascular dementia must be ruled out before making a diagnosis of Alzheimer's.

Vascular dementia is the second leading cause of dementia and must be ruled out when Alzheimer's disease is suspected. There is also a group of psychiatric disorders that can mimic dementia; these disorders, because they are not true dementias, are called pseudodementias. Ordinarily, depression is considered as a pseudodementia when it is severe enough to create symptoms of dementia. In addition, schizophrenia can create symptoms suggestive of dementia. Without adequate personal history, it may be difficult to determine whether symptoms are caused by the thought disorder or dementia. We will discuss vascular dementia in some detail, since it is likely to be considered a potential cause of dementia in initial evaluations. (Depression, another likely candidate related to dementia, is discussed at length in Chapter 3.)

Cumulative effects of several strokes can create dementia.

Most people are familiar with strokes, which cause varying degrees of damage to the brain. The cumulative effects of multiple strokes create dementia by damaging multiple areas of the brain. A single stroke or "infarct" will not usually cause dementia, even though initially this may appear to be the case. However, after the stroke, a person will usually move toward some degree of recovery. With some patients recovery may be partial, but with many recovery can be fairly complete, leaving no significant effects on everyday functioning.

Strokes are caused by blockages in blood vessels or arteries.

The types and severity of strokes vary. Some strokes are caused by blockage of large- or medium-sized blood vessels. Blockage of a large artery can produce massive brain damage, impairing intellectual abilities, voluntary movements, and speech. The brain damage associated with blockage of blood vessels or small arteries may not be so apparent. For instance, the effects of such strokes on intellectual functioning or voluntary movement are so subtle they may not be recognized. Subsequent strokes could occur, involving other small arteries. The cumulative damage of these multiple strokes likely would produce an emerging picture of dementia. When the cumulative effects of small strokes cannot be adequately observed and monitored, it is more difficult to determine whether the dementia is due to multiple small strokes or whether the deterioration of brain functioning is attributable to a primary dementia like Alzheimer's disease.

A single stroke usually results in fairly specific symptoms which do not meet all the criteria for a diagnosis of dementia. Some of the problems caused by strokes include paralysis and restriction of voluntary movement; speech difficulties, ranging from the inability to form words clearly to problems using and comprehending words correctly (expressive and receptive aphasia); emotional instability (moods change rapidly); and impairment of memory or intellectual abilities. When symptoms are pronounced, they will also appear abruptly. If more than one stroke occurs, the deficits will appear to follow a stepwise deteriorating course. One more stroke will occur. Then the affected person will show some progress and improve. If another stroke occurs, other deficits will be evident. Some recovery will take place, but each time another stroke occurs, the overall level of abilities will deteriorate another step. The deficits will not involve all functions of the person initially, but subsequent strokes will create dementia, a vascular dementia.

One kind of stroke is difficult to differentiate from Alzheimer's The results of one type of stroke are very difficult to differentiate from Alzheimer's disease. Called an "angular gyrus syndrome," this kind of stroke involves the brain area supplied with blood and nutrients by the middle cerebral artery (Cummings and Benson 1983). Predisposing medical factors are hypertension or cardiac disease. Aphasia, writing difficulties, calculation deficits, disorientation of right-left sides, and memory problems (actually word-finding difficulties) are some of the symptoms of this kind of stroke. The stroke patient may be apologetic about and frustrated with his language performance; however, the Alzheimer's patient will be unaware of such problems and be more difficult to involve in conversation (Cummings and Benson 1983).

A CAT scan can usually help identify larger stroke damage to the brain. However, small strokes cannot always be detected, which can be the case with the angular gyrus syndrome; often the damaged area is very small.

Vascular dementia must be ruled out before a group of symptoms can indicate an Alzheimer's-type dementia. Sometimes the professionals involved in the evaluation process may have to clearly identify differences in symptoms to make a distinction between Alzheimer's disease and vascular dementia. Laboratory tests, medical history, or even a CAT scan cannot always be helpful in making that distinction.

Even though strokes cause an abrupt appearance of symptoms, a stroke victim may not be aware of the subtle changes caused by a small stroke. Families may be unable to identify such changes in behavior, or they may attribute them to other causes. Strokes are usually painless. They may even occur while the person is sleeping. Early symptoms resulting from some strokes can include dizziness, headaches, and decreased physical and mental vigor. There may be vague physical complaints. Despite the fact strokes can occur suddenly, the onset can be gradual. Such a presentation can be easily confused with Alzheimer's disease. Many times the onset of a stroke is signaled by confusion.

Strokes can have other features that do not necessarily suggest brain damage. The affected individual may demonstrate poor judgment and insight at times. Delirium may occur, and family members may observe hallucinations. Emotional changes may be prevalent. The person who has had a stroke may not exhibit tact or sensitivity in social situations. His concern for others can diminish, and the narrowing of interests in other people and things can lead to increasing self-preoccupation. Depression is not an uncommon consequence for strokes.

Medical conditions create risk for strokes. There are numbers of medical conditions that create risk for strokes. Hypertension, diabetes, and cardiac disease are associated with strokes and vascular dementia. Since strokes are a major cause of death, the suspicion of a stroke should never be treated lightly. If a stroke has occurred, aggressive medical treatment may prevent subsequent strokes, which could lead to a vascular dementia. Additionally, persons known to have Alzheimer's disease can suffer strokes. This possibility is very real; in fact from 20 percent to 25 percent of dementias are caused by a combination of Alzheimer's disease and vascular disease. When it is possible to prevent a stroke or subsequent strokes in an Alzheimer's patient, compounded disabilities can be avoided.

Phases of Alzheimer's Disease

Rate of progressive deterioration varies. Many illnesses follow stages of development and recovery. With Alzheimer's, however, there is no recovery; the slow, progressive course leads to further deterioration of behavior and abilities. For some victims, particularly those under 60, the stages move rapidly, and the illness results in death within three to five years. When the onset begins at a later age, however, the disease may progress slowly for ten years or more.

Understanding of the illness helps adjustment. Both the person who is in the early stages of Alzheimer's and his family naturally want to know what to expect as the illness progresses. An understanding of what is to come allows the family to prepare for future stages, to ease the victim's adjustment, and to gradually accept the disease's effect on the whole family.

Understanding stages helps both families and professionals. The stages of the disease discussed in this chapter are essentially those developed by Dr. Barry Reisberg, Associate Professor of Psychiatry at New York University Medical Center. A general knowledge of these stages can help both families and professionals to do the following:

- Accurately assess and diagnose the condition
- Identify symptoms and follow their progression as the illness develops
- Determine the rate at which the illness is developing
- Have realistic expectations of the patient's capabilities

- Evaluate the adjustment of both family and patient
- Assist family with utilization of appropriate resources.

Manifestations of deficits are dependent upon many factors. Not all Alzheimer's conditions will exactly follow the gradual breakdown indicated in the discussion of stages which follows. There are individual variations that can be attributed to numerous factors: the person's intelligence and abilities before the illness, his personality and basic ways of coping with problems, other health problems, marital relationship, and degree of environmental support.

Stage I: Early Confusional Phase

Forgetfulness becomes a problem. During the beginning stages of Alzheimer's, the patient may seem merely forgetful. As his memory problems worsen, however, the patient's social and occupational skills will begin to diminish noticeably. Although he will usually deny his growing memory problems and successfully compensate at times, he will not be able to catch all of his mistakes.

Confusion and slower responses affect driving. In the early stages, it becomes harder for the person to deal with change and new things. If he travels to an unfamiliar area, he may become lost and confused. However, he probably can still travel familiar routes alone. In traffic, he will be slower to react as his powers of concentration and memory decrease.

Early problems with social conversation surface. During this phase, the person may have trouble finding the right words to communicate his thoughts. Problems in recalling the names of new people and recent conversations may be increasingly apparent. Similarly, he may retain little information from books, magazines, or television shows.

Personality changes appear. The person will begin to lose his spontaneity and sparkle. Socially speaking, he will be slower and less discriminating in what he says and does. His lessened initiative, energy, and drive will be noticeable. He will become more easily upset, anxious, and angry as a result of the uncertainties created by his memory problems. This anxiety, most evident when the person is in demanding social or work-related situations, may cause him to completely avoid unfamiliar or difficult situations.

Denial conceals recognition of early problems. Despite a person's degree of impairment during this early stage, his family may be aware of only a few specific problems. The individual will be using his remaining strengths to cover for his deficits. This denial often leads family members to discount the severity of the person's problems. A person going through the first stages of Alzheimer's disease seems distressed, but the reasons are often a mystery to those closest to him.

Early emotional symptoms are brought to the attention of mental health professionals. At this point, because the symptoms seem to be emotional rather than physical, psychiatrists and other mental health professionals are most likely to be called upon for diagnosis and treatment. Medications might be considered to manage the emotional symptoms. It is important to note that not all persons who exhibit characteristics of the first stage of Alzheimer's disease actually have Alzheimer's. However, if the symptoms of Alzheimer's are present, a diagnosis should be sought, even though it may be distressing to face the full implications of the person's behavior. A victim of Alzheimer's will change gradually but dramatically, and it is both unfair and unrealistic to go on treating the person exactly as in the past.

The disease process results in changes in abilities and actions. It is critical to understand that the Alzheimer's victim's problems are not caused by mere laziness, carelessness, or momentary irrational behavior. The disease is the culprit, and the caregiver must begin to prepare himself for the worsening of problems as the victim slowly declines.

Stage II: Late Confusional Phase

Memory problems are more evident.

As Alzheimer's disease progresses, problems with memory become more evident and somewhat more pervasive. For example, the person's retention of current events declines. He will easily lose the thread of a story and have noticeable difficulties in following conversations. His responses will fail to correspond to the situation. Likewise, his memory of personal history may become foggy.

Decision making and financial management deteriorate.

Making plans or decisions becomes extremely difficult for the person and equally as frustrating for the family. Family members may feel the need to help their relative with his finances and other important responsibilities as it becomes obvious that he is not handling them well.

The denial of problem makes the family's job more difficult.

The affected relative may not welcome assistance. He still may be denying his problems and may see any assistance as interference. The caregiver may see the victim's refusal to admit both his problems and his need for help as impaired judgment. These differences in perception can begin to generate even more conflict within the family. In addition, the victim may choose to avoid social situations altogether as they become too difficult to handle.

Driving becomes riskier.

The person's driving also becomes a source of concern. At this stage, the Alzheimer's patient probably can travel familiar routes with reasonable safety. However, he is vulnerable to mistakes and improper responses to unforeseen situations. He may overreact or not react at all to potentially dangerous traffic conditions. The family should seriously consider curtailing or eliminating driving opportunities.

Orientation in time and place is affected. Some aspects of the person's memory—his orientation to time, place, and person—may still be intact at this stage. However, his difficulties in concentrating may make it difficult to recall these things or to recall the events of the past few minutes or the past week. On the other hand, memories of the distant past can be surprisingly clear and accurate. He may speak more often about past events and avoid conversations about current events.

Supervision means supportive assistance. The Alzheimer's victim will need some supervision and daily support during this stage. Although he is not disabled in all aspects of his life, he will need help in more complex areas such as handling his finances and paying his bills. The mixture of stress and detailed organization necessary to file income tax reports, balance a checkbook, and pay bills may be more than he can handle.

The victim becomes self-absorbed and depressed. As the victim sees his capabilities slipping away, he is likely to become increasingly self-absorbed and insensitive to the feelings of others. Often, the victim sinks into depression, making his situation even worse. The caregiver, trying to assist a loved one with problems he denies having, can easily feel rejected and unappreciated.

Stage III: Early Dementia

Dependency increases the caregiver's load. By this time, the Alzheimer's victim has become quite dependent on others for his care. That dependency increases the caregiver's sense of responsibility for meeting all of the person's needs and keeping him safe from harm. It is difficult for someone who is not involved in the actual care to understand how much must be done daily. In fact, other family members may fail to support the primary caregiver because they cannot envision how strenuous the mental and physical demands of daily caregiving are. A person in the early dementia phase requires:

- Help in initiating most activities
- Someone to help him "think"
- "Hands-on" care as his dependencies increase
- Help in expressing his needs.

The victim should not drive. A person who is exhibiting symptoms of early dementia is a hazardous driver. For example, he may increase his speed or drive through stop signs unknowingly. Likewise, stressful situations encountered while driving can dramatically affect his judgment. Family members therefore must take it upon themselves to ensure that the patient does not drive.

Memory gaps trigger insecurity and defensive behavior. Even though his problems are obvious to everyone around, the patient may continue to deny and shield his mistakes. In conversations he may fabricate information that seems irrelevant or absurd. Actually, he is valiantly trying to fill in information gaps created by memory loss. The patient is trying to pull together pieces of his own reality in order to maintain a meaningful life.

As his memory deteriorates, a heightened sense of insecurity can develop into suspicion and paranoia. Judgment and reasoning deteriorate further. His suspiciousness may be accompanied by anger, even when a family member tries to prove his accusations or suspicions are unfounded. Agitated behavior may develop.

Emotional reactions become more prominent. The patient's emotional instability comes from a mixture of psychological, social, and neurological sources. During this stage, the Alzheimer's patient may have periodic crying spells and abrupt mood changes, with or without obvious causes. Such instability can be frightening and aggravating to families. Soothing, calming approaches that convey support and understanding are good responses on the caregiver's part.

Memory deficits fluctuate. Fluctuations in memory on an almost moment-to-moment basis are not uncommon in Stage III. Caregivers should realize that such fluctuations are a normal part of the disease, making the best of those days when their relative seems better, and avoiding despondency when he seems worse.

Logical, sequential reasoning and actions diminish. The victim's ability to recall the correct sequences of behavior and tasks becomes seriously impaired. This inability may show up in areas such as dressing or grooming, where he may complete only part of the task.

Independence encouraged Usually, he can continue to perform part of his daily routine with help. It is easy, however, to increase his dependency unnecessarily by assuming certain things are too intricate for him to complete. For example, by Stage III he will need help in selecting properly matched and appropriate clothing, but this does not mean he cannot still dress himself. Some persons with Alzheimer's will want to wear the same clothes every day, without changing or washing them. Although this kind of behavior will tempt caregivers to take over the entire task, the patient should be encouraged to care for himself as long as possible.

Simple decisions become overwhelming. During early dementia, a person will have difficulty making even simple decisions concerning eating or dressing. But the caregiver still can offer simple alternatives that require a yes or no response. It may be helpful to suggest a choice of two necessary alternatives, such as bathing or picking up the dirty clothes. This increases the chance that the patient will undertake at least one desirable course of action.

**Social with-
drawal is
accompanied
by impaired
thinking
capacity.**
The affected person can be expected to withdraw
from both social and task-oriented activities. His
decreasing thinking and reasoning abilities will
make him less flexible and able to adjust to stressful situations. If he is pushed, he will become both
overly anxious and angry; if he is pushed too often,
he will refuse to do even necessary stressful activi-
ties. Nonetheless, he may still enjoy some social situations. For example, going to church or the movies may still be fairly undemanding,
while visiting with long-time friends may be overwhelming.

**Caregivers re-
quire support.**
At this point, caregivers need considerable
emotional support and relief from their full-time
responsibilities. Family members, friends, and
neighbors can provide both the support and the
relief the primary caregiver needs, whether it is by sitting with the
relative, doing chores, or visiting. Caregivers should carefully monitor their own ability to handle the demands placed upon them, and
they should not hesitate to ask for help as needed.

Stage IV:　Middle Dementia

**The victim
reacts more
severely to
loss of
abilities.**
Major changes occur as the disease progresses from early to middle dementia, and the
involvement of caregivers increases considerably. Throughout the illness, the patient may
have been fairly successful in using denial to
protect himself from the realization that his
mind is slipping away. However, denial is becoming a less effective
protector. Withdrawal is being replaced by tendencies toward agitation, paranoia, and delusions. The need for security cannot be satisfied by the victim's mind. At this point, the environment can meet
this need through structure, routine, and caring.

Delusions
Delusions often reflect fears of loss and imagined
threats in the external world. Spouses may be

accused of being unfaithful. Neighbors and friends may be blamed for unbelievable things.

**Sleep distur-
bances and
hallucinations**

During this phase, the patient's sleep is more often disrupted and erratic. He may be awakened by hallucinations or delusional fears that make it almost impossible to sleep, and he may begin to wander at night.

**Repetitive
behavior**

A number of emotional changes appear during the middle dementia stage. They may include compulsive symptoms such as pulling clothes out of drawers and replacing them over and over. The person may not be able to hold onto his thoughts long enough to complete a course of action. Obsessive thoughts or repetitive ideas and concerns may be more evident in some persons.

**Movement and
coordination
difficulties**

The victim's problems with movement and coordination may become more obvious now and interfere markedly with his performance. He will develop difficulties with walking and with the purposeful, coordinated movements required for dressing, eating, brushing his teeth, and so forth. Eating difficulties may contribute to weight loss; alternatively, excessive eating may become a problem.

**Help with daily
activities is
essential.**

At this point, the Alzheimer's victim requires assistance with most activities of daily living. The caregiver must carefully and sensitively adjust his social and behavioral expectations of the patient downward. The individual must not be placed in situations that could lead to emotional overload; he could overreact in violent and frightening ways.

**Sources of vi-
olent behavior**

Much of the violent behavior of persons with Alzheimer's disease is triggered by excessive environmental demands. The person is unable to comprehend what behavior is expected of him and may respond inappropriately. Pressure to respond to situations promptly further accentuates inappropriate responses. Too many choices or options can precipitate more anxiety and agitation or may lead to further withdrawal.

Bathing problems emerge. The middle dementia stage brings a real fear of bathing. This fear is often misinterpreted by caregivers as simple stubbornness and uncooperativeness. But actually, the person's fear of bathing is related to reasonable concerns. The patient forgets how to adjust water temperature and how to use the soap and washcloth. His impaired coordination creates difficulties in getting in and out of the tub, and he may fear falling. In addition, the patient has lost his sense of the social importance of personal hygiene. To reduce conflict over bathing, the caregiver may substitute towel washing for a tub bath or reduce the frequency of bathing. Sometimes the patient may accept a hot bath as a way to relieve tensions, especially when it is combined with a soothing body massage.

Loss of touch with events and experiences Persons in middle dementia are generally unaware of their surroundings, the time of year, the year itself, and other indications of time and place. Memory abilities deteriorate to a fragmentary knowledge of home address and whereabouts. Getting lost becomes almost inevitable and is a real worry for caregivers. The patient may be able to distinguish strangers from familiar persons, but often he cannot identify the person on whom he is most dependent, his spouse. He will usually know his own name and have some sketchy recall of his past, but he is largely unaware of all recent events and experiences. He may give pieces of information which have no clear meaning. For the victim of Alzheimer's, the world has become frightening and largely unmanageable. The loss of cognitive, memory, and perceptual abilities prevents him from organizing the pieces of his life into a meaningful whole.

Caregiving becomes lonelier and more isolating. At this stage, caregiving takes up most of the day and night, yet the caregiver receives little or no recognition from the patient. Kindness is rarely seen, unless it is read into some small action or gesture. This is extremely difficult for many caregivers to accept, since they naturally seek gratitude and approval from their relative.

If the caregiver has assumed solitary care for the victim, he is likely to become severely isolated, both physically and socially. Friends no longer visit, and community activities are restricted. The greatest isolation is created by the inability of the victim to relate to the caregiver spouse. All decisions fall on his shoulders. There are no rewards and appreciation for the caregiving, unless the caregiver finds ways to affirm himself and compensate for the emotional isolation and separation.

Caregiver must hire help or place the victim in an institution. By this stage, the emotional burdens of caregiving force those involved to make difficult decisions about whether to hire in-home help or possibly place the person in an institution. In Stage IV, hiring full-time assistance is the ideal situation for caregivers. However, it is costly to hire experienced full-time help; thus part-time help may be the best alternative. But the primary caregiver must have some relief from the consuming tasks of direct care and supervision. In addition, the patient may need some form of psychiatric or other professional mental health assistance.

Caregivers need support groups. Even with help, the caregiver's role may become so demanding as to totally overwhelm his life. The patient's sleeping problems are likely to disrupt the caregiver's sleep; his agitation makes management more perplexing and tiring; his delusional beliefs are painful and frightening. A family support group can help. The caregiver may also feel a need for individual counseling and assistance in securing other supportive resources.

The caregiver should call upon the whole family for help and support as needed. Major decisions regarding other arrangements for the patient's final weeks, months, or years are forthcoming, and few caregivers should be making such decisions without some degree of family input and support.

When family members do not support the most appropriate course of action, the primary caregiver must be reassured by others that he is making the correct decisions. Conflicts may develop because relatives do not understand the implications of the illness and the daily strains of caregiving.

Stage V: Late Dementia

Such phrases as "a long good-bye" or an "unending death" have been used to describe the disease's final stage. Caregivers must give so much for so small a response that often all the questions of life seem to be best summed up in one word—"WHY?"

Recognize limitations of caregiving. Decisions now must be made without the loved one's nod of approval. Notions of what is best or what he would have wanted compete with the fact that one must decide alone. As narrow as the victim's life has become, it is still valuable to the family, and it is hard to say good-bye. Nonetheless, one hopes to see the suffering end. Although the caregiver may want to keep his loved one at home, an institution may be the only realistic alternative when he can no longer provide full-time care.

Denial may continue to protect the victim from the emotional impact of the illness. He may still be able to smile, to laugh, and to appear to enjoy life at times.

There is less of everything. The emotional experience of life can go on even though the words have been lost. Behaviorally, the person is as likely to be amenable as he is to be difficult. The need for tranquilizers lessens because his behavior has become more easily managed.

His motor abilities will continue to deteriorate and eventually his ability to walk, sit, and smile will be lost, as well as his control of bladder and colon functions. The loss may be uneven: a person who is still walking may be found on the floor or caught as he falls because he suddenly has forgotten how to walk. Such cases may require medical attention to ensure that a stroke or transient ischemic attack (condition in which blood supply to the brain is temporarily interrupted) has not occurred.

Addressing movement problems
It is important to help the Alzheimer's victim to walk as long as he is able. He will not be able to use a walker, since he has lost his coordination, but guardrails and other supports can help. In addition, rearranging furniture to provide support and eliminating barriers (such as loose rugs) will help the individual in his walking. The use of geriatric chairs and other confining devices should be avoided as much as possible; such confinement increases agitation and restlessness.

Eating difficulties
During this final stage, the patient will eventually lose the ability to chew and swallow food. The caregiver may have to cut the food into small pieces or prepare an almost totally soft diet. If the patient refuses to eat, other methods of feeding must be considered.

Need more structured, highly supervised care
As brain activity becomes severely disturbed, the patient is increasingly vulnerable to seizures as well as aspiration, pneumonia, infection, and other illnesses. He will need assistance in eating, since choking, blockage, or other problems in breathing and swallowing can occur. Respiratory problems can worsen through decreased activity, particularly when the person becomes bedridden.

The final reconciliation
Stupor occurs in this terminal stage and leads finally to coma and death. Throughout the illness, the caregiver has had to meet one challenge after another in caring for his loved one. Human

contact has made a real difference to the Alzheimer's victim. Such contact is still important, even if the person is seemingly unable to respond. Patience and kindness, though they require great strength, are necessary. A touch, a loving voice, and the presence of a loved one help keep a person physically and emotionally alive, even when he can no longer reach out to anyone.

3

DEPRESSION AND ALZHEIMER'S

Depression is a serious psychiatric condition. Although we commonly use the term "depressed" to describe someone who is feeling down or out-of-sorts, severe depression is actually a serious psychiatric condition. Unlike the temporary moodiness that is normal to daily life, clinical depression is not a condition that one recovers from easily, although the condition can be cured. Because depression often accompanies Alzheimer's disease, it is important that caregivers learn to recognize the condition and seek treatment for symptoms.

Symptoms of depression Depression is a prolonged disturbance of mood that colors a person's whole inner perception of the world. She feels down in the dumps, unworthy, and may feel that life is not worth living. The symptoms of depression include feelings of sadness and emptiness, withdrawal from others, self-neglect, sleeping problems, and many other emotional and physical signs, which are listed in more detail later in this chapter. Because many of these same symptoms also accompany Alzheimer's disease, it is easy for depression to go unrecognized and untreated in an Alzheimer's patient.

Professional help should be sought. If caregivers suspect that their loved one is seriously depressed, they should not hesitate to seek psychiatric treatment, which can be quite beneficial. In a few cases, a patient suffering from depression may even have been diagnosed mistakenly as having Alzheimer's. It is therefore important that a check for depression be made as part of the diagnostic work-up for all patients suffering from an Alzheimer's-type dementia.

Depression is more likely in the early stages.

A person with Alzheimer's is most likely to suffer from severe depression during the earlier stages of the illness, when she still has the faculties to comprehend the full implications of the disease. The disturbing changes she is experiencing naturally lead her to become depressed about the future, but her depression in turn may intensify the effects of the disease.

Risk factors for depression

Persons who have previously suffered from depression are at a particular risk of becoming depressed in the face of Alzheimer's. Also at risk are highly achievement-oriented and perfectionist personalities. Difficult social and family situations can trigger depression, particularly when the victim lacks any source of emotional support. In other cases depression may be brought on simply by reduced self-esteem or loss of income caused by Alzheimer's. Denial of this illness may not be sufficient protection from what is happening.

Symptoms of depression are hard to recognize in an Alzheimer's victim.

The symptoms of depression can be hard to isolate and recognize when Alzheimer's is present although they should be evident to a mental health professional. Often a close evaluation is required to determine whether Alzheimer's or depression or both are causing a particular behavior. For example, the urge to withdraw from social situations could indicate either condition, but reasons may be different.

Depression characterized by a number of symptoms

Like dementia, depression is characterized by a cluster of symptoms. Although none of these symptoms is necessarily significant alone, when they exist in combination for an extended period of time, a severe depression may be indicated.

Physical symptoms of depression

Numerous physical complaints that cannot be explained by any known medical problem may indicate depression. Such physical symptoms include:

- Weakness, unexplained fatigue, dizzy spells, low energy
- Gastrointestinal problems such as pain, indigestion, constipation
- Urinary disturbances
- Changes in eating habits, appetite, and weight
- Loss of sexual desire
- Sleeping disturbances, including awakening during the night or early morning awakening
- Slowed movement or more agitated movement
- Slowed speech; softened, lowered, or monotone voice; incomplete responses.

Psychological symptoms of depression

Depression also brings on a whole range of psychological symptoms. These may include:

- Tension, anxiety, and irritability
- Loss of initiative and interest
- Indecisiveness and ambivalence
- Inability to take pleasure in favorite activities
- Apathy, boredom, indifference, and resisting activity
- Doing little or nothing ·
- Loss of interest in grooming and personal care
- Poor attention and concentration
- Extreme sensitivity to problems with memory
- Excessive complaints and worries
- Tendency to cry and get upset over little things.

Guilt, suicidal ideas, sense of inadequacy, and hopelessness

Other common symptoms associated with depression include expressions of guilt and concern about making up for perceived wrongs done to others or omissions of responsibilities toward family and friends. Preoccupations with death and suicidal ideas or the desire to die occur in more serious depression. In earlier stages of Alzheimer's, the depressed person's suicidal ideas must be taken particularly seriously. Feelings of failure, inadequacy, helplessness, and powerlessness all characterize the low self-evaluation of a depressed person. An underlying dementia further stimulates and reinforces such views. Negative expectations, self-blame, and self-criticism can reinforce each other to create a downward emotional spiral.

Seek professional help for depression.
Many depressed persons deny some of the emotional symptoms of the illness or have difficulty reporting them. Should symptoms characteristic of depression be noted during the progression of Alzheimer's, caregivers need to seek professional help. Some of these symptoms could be suggestive of an ongoing grief process, but this should be evaluated by a professional familiar with depression. Treatment of depression is important, for it can improve both the person's outlook and functioning.

Caregivers also suffer from depression.
Caregivers may recognize some of the symptoms described here developing in themselves. Though these may be brought on by grief or stress rather than clinical depression, caregivers who experience the symptoms of depression should consult a mental health professional. Caring for an Alzheimer's patient is difficult enough without the added burden of a severe depression.

A case example: The impact depression has in Alzheimer's disease.
Harry Sims, a 54-year-old male, came to our center one day with his wife Julie who was 47 years old. Recently, Harry had learned he had Alzheimer's disease. It had been diagnosed at a major medical center. He made light of his diagnosis because his principal concern was his wife's adjustment to the illness. They had only been married for five years and her 13-year-old son lived in the household. Harry had a business of his own.

Julie had helped with the business, but her husband had always been in total control of everything he did. He was also a perfectionist, and her work had never been remotely acceptable to him. His strong personality was a definite contrast to her own. She was reserved and reticent. Julie had serious doubts about her abilities, and her self-esteem was quite low. Her husband's illness was frightening to her.

She was equally apprehensive about their financial future. She questioned how long Harry could continue to handle the business. His solution to this was to have her run the business or find someone else that he could trust to run it with his assistance. Harry had very high expectations of his wife, and he would put great pressure on any other person who became responsible for the business. It was more significant that Harry placed even greater pressure on himself.

Mr. Sims' concerns about his wife's adjustment to the illness translated into his concerns about the family business. His lack of confidence in his wife heightened his insecurity about this matter. He seemed to project any of his shortcomings onto his wife. This had worsened over the past year and created considerable tension between the couple. Another sore point concerned Julie's son. He could not walk the line for his stepfather, and the two battled constantly. This was a matter of great distress for Julie who seemed to be stuck in the middle.

Over a period of several weeks the couple came for counseling. They were able to make some improvements. Julie, particularly, began to appreciate what was beginning to happen to her husband. Nevertheless, tensions continued to build. Harry became progressively more hostile and verbally aggressive. They stayed in separate parts of their home and no longer had meals together. The conflict between Harry and his stepson escalated. Over one weekend, tempers flared, and the situation exploded; the wife and her son left the house and stayed with friends.

On Monday of the following week they came to our center in separate cars. Our psychiatrist saw both, and medication was given on a trial basis to reduce Harry's extreme agitation and hostile behavior. After two weeks, it appeared the situation had improved somewhat. This was partly attributable to the fact that Julie's son had gone to live with a brother and his family.

Julie was having as difficult a time as Harry in her own way. When she and Harry were seen together, it was clear that she was suffering from clinical depression. Her appetite was poor, and she was not sleeping well at night. Her ability to concentrate and remember was affected. She experienced extreme anxiety and was apprehensive of her husband much of the time. Her energy level was very low, and fatigue had become a constant complaint. Stomach distress was a major physical complaint. Her low self-esteem was even lower and she had helpless and hopeless feelings. It was terrible to consider the future. She was given an antidepressant medication.

Considerable improvement was noted when she and her husband came again in two weeks. Their relationship had improved slightly. She was having more contact with her few friends. This had been a recommendation because she was isolated. Harry had few friends himself and had initially controlled her contact with the few friends they did have. They lived 10 miles outside a small rural city, which accentuated the sense of isolation and loneliness that Julie experienced.

Several factors were considered before Harry and Julie returned for their next appointment. First, Harry had a very high need for control which he was losing. His wife had become a liability as his own denial of the illness failed to protect him. He had often stated that he could handle the Alzheimer's disease. It became clear that his attempts to get help for his wife were actually attempts to get help for himself. The security of remaining life was dependent upon someone else. Before, Harry had not been able to depend upon or trust anyone.

Harry had never demonstrated any of the memory impairment typical of Alzheimer's disease. Few people would have believed that he could have Alzheimer's disease. The major effect of the illness was on his speech. His speech was pressured and circumlocutory. He tended to repeat himself a little. There was a problem in expressing ideas clearly, and Harry admitted he had trouble getting his thoughts together. Nevertheless, he demonstrated skillful compensations for any underlying deficits. The agitation and low tolerance for frustration created the biggest problem in his business. He got too easily upset with his customers and became overwhelmed more easily by work demand.

There was reasonable doubt in some minds about whether he actually had Alzheimer's disease, but the medical center had been thorough in its evaluation. We began to suspect that he was suffering from depression. He complained some about fatigue and concentration, both of which are not uncommon in Alzheimer's disease. However, Harry usually denied having any significant problems with memory. There were many more somatic complaints. He had a distracting ringing in his ears and experienced some pain in his legs. He had stomach distress and complained of headaches. Tension, anxiety, and agitation were quite evident.

Harry's personality style provided other clues. He had some paranoid tendencies that were consistent with the controlling, compulsive traits. It was significant that he had few friends and did not form relationships easily. In fact, he was somewhat aloof and seldom spoke in a language of feelings. This all led to the conclusion that we were dealing with a masked depression that was associated with agitation. It was somatically characterized.

An antidepressant medication was prescribed, and the medication for the agitation was discontinued. Careful monitoring of the medication revealed no significant side effects. The only complaint was a dry mouth. A remarkable change was observed in a very short time. In two weeks this husband and wife reported that their relationship was better than it had ever been. As treatment continued, Harry began to voice the nightmare he had been living before the antidepressant was given. His fears about the illness surfaced, and we were able to deal with these feelings. He also showed that he was aware of how destructive his role in the family had become. He swallowed a great deal of pride to indicate that he had been wrong about some things, including mistakes with his stepson.

Harry and Julie began to find pleasure and enjoyment in their lives again. Harry was more accepting of his wife and other people. They were able to move to a smaller rent house they owned in town. This afforded them the opportunity to have more social contact. Harry was aware that the medication actually helped clear his thinking some. All of the somatic complaints were gone within the first two weeks.

This story began seven months ago. Harry exhibits some slight deterioration (visual-spatial problems, memory, and abstract reasoning), but some major issues are resolved. The business is presently being operated by him and his wife. His expectations are more realistic. The other critical change makes an even greater difference. The relationship with Julie's son has been reestablished, and the couple has more involvement with their respective families.

Our example above illustrates several points. First, it may be quite difficult to distinguish depression from Alzheimer's disease, particularly in some individuals and situations. Secondly, both the suspected Alzheimer's patient and caregiver spouse can be depressed. The nature of their respective coping styles can aggravate the situation even more. Depression itself is strengthened. Finally, old conflicts that have been largely unresolved can surface in such stressful caregiving situations. The needs and problems of all family members must be considered in treatment.

Recognizing and treating depression with Alzheimer's disease is a very significant intervention. Caregivers may be prone to develop depression or serious reactions to continuous stress. For this reason professionals must carefully consider how family caregivers are coping with the physical, emotional, and social aspects of the disease. Support and learning new ways to deal effectively with the demands of caregiving can be helpful, but depression may require other treatment approaches such as antidepressant medications.

4

POSSIBLE CAUSES OF ALZHEIMER'S DISEASE

Background to research

Many clues to Alzheimer's disease have been identified, but the different trails down which these leads have taken us have yet to converge on any single explanation of one cause. There is a growing belief that Alzheimer's is a disease that is caused by many factors, and that these factors must act in some sequence or combination for the disease to be expressed. The abnormal protein beta amyloid, for example, is associated with a genetic cause of the disease, and it is implicated in causing the death of neurons. Some believe it has a very important central and precipitating role in the development of the disease, though its exact role remains a topic of investigation.

Of the causes being considered, genetic factors are the only ones that have been proven to account for the disease in a small percentage of cases. Genetic factors will be discussed in some detail. Theories concerning slow viruses, the immune system and brain inflammation, and excessive aluminum will also be discussed.

It also appears highly likely that certain psychosocial factors can contribute to when Alzheimer's disease develops and the apparent severity of its symptoms. We therefore will look at the possible relevancy for Alzheimer's of such psychosocial factors as environment, psychiatric history, social and sensory deprivation, and one's sense of support and control.

What does not cause Alzheimer's

A word also seems in order about what does NOT cause Alzheimer's disease. It is not caused by simple old age, hardening of the arteries, or stroke. Most importantly, it is not caused by the person's character or behavior. "Bad" or "lazy" people do not develop Alzheimer's disease any more often than "good" people. No one has ever "deserved" to get Alzheimer's disease. Although caregivers and others struggling to understand the inexplicable may be tempted to create such explanations, perhaps subconsciously, it can only make a difficult situation unnecessarily harder to imagine that the victim or anyone else is to blame for the disease. The seemingly "crazy" behavior of an Alzheimer's victim is brought about by very real physical and chemical changes in the brain (see Chapter 14) over which the person can have no control. Let us hope the true causes of these changes and of the disease itself can be identified soon.

The Genetic Theory

Genes and genetic factors linked to Alzheimer's disease

Genes and genetic factors have significant roles in Alzheimer's disease. Evidence today links genes on five chromosomes—1, 12, 14, 19, and 21—to the disease. Less than ten years ago, chromosome 21 held much of the interest of those conducting genetic research. Very recently, researchers have found evidence of a new gene for late-onset Alzheimer's on chromosome 12 (Stephenson 1997). Genetic factors were already known to have a part in the development of other brain diseases. Huntington's chorea and Down's syndrome are two examples. Alzheimer's disease and Down's syndrome have several features in common. The amyloid plaques and neurofibrillary tangles that occur in Alzheimer's disease are found in the brain tissue of individuals with Down's syndrome. Individuals with Down's syndrome invariably develop Alzheimer's disease if they live past age 40. There are extra copies of chromosome 21 in Down's syndrome victims. This association of Alzheimer's with chromosome 21 has hastened genetic inquiry.

Familial Alzheimer's is linked to chromosome 21. Subsequent research has shown that a genetic defect on chromosome 21 accounts for a pattern of genetic transmission known as autosomal-dominant inheritance in a very small number of families with early-onset Alzheimer's disease (St. George-Hyslop, Tanzi, et al. 1987). This indicates that 50 percent of first-degree relatives (parents, brothers or sisters, and children) would develop the disease if the type of genetic expression is complete penetrance. The defect on chromosome 21 also includes a gene that is involved in the formation of the abnormal amyloid protein.

Familial and sporadic cases Chromosomal links have been sought to explain other family pedigrees in which the disease seemed to be following some pattern of inheritance. A small number of families with some type of inheritance pattern affecting several generations have been identified around the world. In addition to chromosome 21, autosomal-dominant patterns of inheritance have been linked to chromosomes 1 and 14. The familial form of Alzheimer's disease seems to be caused by inheritance of gene mutations linked to these chromosomes. Chromosome 14 has the gene mutation that accounts for most of the familial cases of Alzheimer's disease. These familial cases account for about 5 percent of the disease; the remaining 95 percent are sporadic with seemingly random occurrence (Roses 1996). Most familial cases are early-onset, but findings connected with a gene mutation on chromosome 19 identified both an increased risk for the common, late-onset Alzheimer's disease (Corder et al. 1993) and a protein (apolipoprotein E) that binds to beta-amyloid. The gene on chromosome 12 is also thought to increase a person's susceptibility.

ApoE genes The most common form of Alzheimer's disease, late-onset (age 65 and older), has some familial but mainly sporadic types. From 50 to 75 percent of late-onset cases are associated with the inheritance of various forms of the apolipoprotein E (apoE) gene, already well-known as a carrier of cholesterol in the blood, found on chromosome 19 (Roses 1996). There are three forms, or alleles, of this gene—apoE2, apoE3, and apoE4. ApoE3 is the most common form in the general population; more than 50 percent of the population have a matched pair of the apoE3 allele. ApoE4 increases the risk of developing Alzheimer's. People who inherit two apoE4 genes—one from the father and one from the mother—are at least eight times more likely to develop the disease than persons who have two of the more common apoE3 allele. Having one or two of the E4 allele seems to also influence the age at which symptoms develop. The least common allele, apoE2, may actually lower the risk for developing Alzheimer's disease. New findings indicate that apoE4 is not a risk factor for late-onset cases past 70 (Stephenson 1997), thus reducing the percentage of late-onset cases influenced by the apoE4 gene.

Genetic screening   ApoE4 is a risk factor for developing Alzheimer's disease. Developing screening tests to identify persons at risk for developing Alzheimer's on the basis of apoE status on a broad basis is tempting. Predictive testing is possible for the autosomal-dominant genes. However, apoE status cannot tell whether or not someone will get Alzheimer's disease. Some people with the gene do not develop Alzheimer's; others without it do. Having an E4 allele doesn't foretell disease unless one has symptoms. Genetic factors provide the basis for understanding some of the ways Alzheimer's disease develops. Even these, however, do not account for that many cases, and some of the most compelling facts fail to converge on one path toward any single theory of cause. Findings surrounding the identification of APP (amyloid precursor protein) and apoE4 genes have created excitement, yet not everyone with these develops Alzheimer's. Other genes, as yet unidentified, are likely to explain more of the puzzle concerning causes of the disease—why some develop it and others don't. Other undetermined factors must act as triggers for the development of the disease, interacting with genetic factors.

The Viral Theory

An extremely slow infectious virus may be the cause. Another theory holds that Alzheimer's disease is caused by an extremely slow, infectious virus that may take several decades to incubate. Other neurological disorders have been found to be caused by such viruses; these include Kuru, Creutzfeldt-Jakob disease, and Gerstmann-Straussler syndrome (Prusiner 1984). These viruses are similar to a viral agent that causes the neurological disorder, scrapie, in sheep and goats. This infectious agent, a prion, is much smaller than conventional viruses.

It has never been shown that Alzheimer's can be transmitted. To prove that such a virus for Alzheimer's disease exists, clinical studies would have to show that the disease can be transmitted. So far, laboratory tests attempting to transmit the disease from brain tissue to animals have failed. It may be, however, that the animals simply were not susceptible to the disease or that the incubation period for the disease is longer than the duration of the studies (Prusiner 1984). (Kuru and Creutzfeldt-Jakob disease, for example, are known to incubate for 20–30 years.) Such a long incubation period would seem consistent with the late age onset usually found in Alzheimer's.

Some studies have explored the theory that Alzheimer's is caused by a combination of viral and familial/genetic factors. Others have suggested a relationship between amyloid plaques and viral-like agents. Since no hard evidence exists to either confirm or deny the idea that Alzheimer's is caused by a virus, this theory must remain an active area for further research.

The Immune-System Theory

Increasing chronological age is the strongest risk factor for Alzheimer's disease. The elderly tend to get more autoimmune diseases such as cancer, late-onset diabetes, and rheumatoid arthritis (Nee

1983). Other neurological diseases—including multiple sclerosis and Huntington's chorea—are known to involve immune system alterations; several studies report findings suggesting abnormalities of brain immune function that may contribute to the progression of Alzheimer's disease (Peskind 1996). Loss of neurons and the appearance of plaques and tangles may be partly mediated by the immune system (Rogers et al. 1992). There is now considerable evidence that the Alzheimer's disease brain suffers a chronic inflammatory state. This is not the inflammation we associate with a wound; it refers to the primary reactions characteristic of the brain's immune response. The possibility exists that an immune system attack might be responsible for much of the neuronal destruction in Alzheimer's disease (McGeer and McGeer 1996). The finding that nonsteroidal anti-inflammatory drugs might decrease the risk of developing Alzheimer's (Breitner and Gau et al. 1994) lends additional support to the suggestion that altered brain immune function is somehow involved. Even with evidence that the basic processes of immune response and inflammation can be observed in the Alzheimer's brain, one important question remains. Do immune mechanisms in this disease merely reflect natural processes to help the damaged brain heal, or might these mechanisms be a source of damage (Rogers et al. 1992)?

The Aluminum Theory

High levels of aluminum in the brain may cause Alzheimer's. Some researchers have theorized that neurofibrillary tangles in Alzheimer's disease and other dementias could be caused by an excess of aluminum in the brain. The concentration of aluminum in the human brain is known to increase with age (Yates 1979; Jenike 1985). Abnormally high levels of aluminum have been found in the brains of persons suffering from other dementias (Thienhaus 1985), though these may well be unrelated to the disease. Together these indications suggest that high levels of aluminum may possibly be related to Alzheimer's disease, though there is certainly no proof of its being a causative factor.

Chelation therapy not proven helpful
Some health practitioners advertise chelation therapy and imply that this therapy will reduce aluminum levels and thus improve the impairments that characterize Alzheimer's disease. There is simply no scientific support for this idea. Often such clinics fail to properly diagnose Alzheimer's disease, assuming that the patient's problems are caused by treatable "vascular dementia." Since chelation therapy is expensive, can produce serious side effects, and has never been proved to help Alzheimer's patients, such treatment should be discouraged. Too often it simply drains the pocketbooks of families desperate for a cure.

Concern about aluminum has led many families to worry about the risks of using aluminum cookware and aluminum-rich antacids and other medications. Though there is no evidence that prolonged use of these products affects Alzheimer's in any way, some researchers suggest that concerned families may wish to request medications with less aluminum from their doctors (Shore and Wyatt 1983) when their medications are extremely high in aluminum.

Psychosocial Factors and Dementia

Negative psychosocial factors create obstacles to caregiving and adjustment.
Psychosocial factors can have powerful effects, both positive and negative, on the lives of people. On the positive side, such things as an adequate income, consistent family support, and a comfortable home environment make caring for a person with dementia much less burdensome. On the negative side, serious health problems, excessive family conflicts, and the absence of daily routines can create obstacles in the care of and adjustment to Alzheimer's disease. Viewed in this context, psychosocial factors can have a definite relationship to how a person with alzheimer's disease will fare in the long run.

In addition, feelings about the causes of the disease can influence both the caregiver's attitudes and those of the family toward Alzheimer's patients. Family members sometimes wonder whether there is anything in their relative's history that could have caused or contributed to his condition. Family members sometimes blame severe, recent illnesses for precipitating symptoms of dementia. However, if their relative's condition meets criteria for Alzheimer's disease, these other medical problems will have already been ruled out as the cause of the dementia.

Medical trauma can precipitate symptoms. We have seen a few cases in which the aftermath of traumatic medical conditions or reactions to severe losses or psychosocial stressors seem to contribute to the progression of Alzheimer's disease.

Sometimes, a person traumatized by serious medical conditions will begin to exhibit symptoms of dementia. Usually, these symptoms preceded the illness in a very subtle form, but become more pronounced afterwards. Additionally, unlike the hospital-type delirium that occurs with older persons, these symptoms do not disappear. In fact, the person's intellectual and memory abilities not only fail to return but continue to deteriorate. These medical conditions do not cause Alzheimer's disease; they simply precipitate a worsening of the process.

Reactions to the loss of a spouse can hide symptoms of dementia. In the case of reactions to losses or other stressors, the most common situation is the loss of a spouse. Prior to the spouse's death, the surviving spouse will often seem to be handling things relatively well, considering the demands of care and the emotional adjustment. Any subtle symptoms of dementia can be explained as normal reactions to the circumstances. We have also seen cases where the medically ill spouse was the "cognitive" manager of the care situation. He or she kept household activities, bills, and medications under control. These persons, even though physically ill, were caregivers in a sense for the spouse who was later found to have an Alzheimer's-type dementia. When this significant other dies or goes to a nursing home, the spouse left at home may experience substantial loss of organization, routine, and support. Grief and/or depression may be observed.

The grief or depression may not immediately appear, but it may emerge later as reactions to coping with dramatic life changes. It may be difficult initially to determine whether the impairments of memory and intellectual abilities are the symptoms of dementia or reactions to what has happened. Pseudodementia may be present in the form of depression, which can coexist with Alzheimer's disease.

Medical problems and significant psychosocial losses can enhance the symptoms of Alzheimer's disease. Again, these events do not cause the disease; they accentuate symptoms that were already developing insidiously.

No connection between past events and Alzheimer's disease   Families sometimes try to blame psychosocial stressors or other past events in a person's life for Alzheimer's disease, even though there is no connection. Relatives' beliefs at times center on things that should or should not have been done (e.g., he should have worked harder, or he worked too hard). Family members may point to some specific event in the past that brought about changes in their relative's behavior. For example, they may say their relative never was the same after his parents died or after he lost a job 15 years ago or after he had a knock-down-drag-out fight with his brother. They may try to resurrect these problems as explanations for Alzheimer's disease. Behavioral changes, indeed, may have occurred in their relative after these kinds of events, yet there is no reason to believe these events cause the degenerative brain disease.

When a person affected by Alzheimer's disease has had a troubled life long before the illness began, there may be considerable hard feelings and conflicts within his family. Family members may be both bitter and resentful of things they believe their affected relative did to them or others. In this case, what the family says is the cause for Alzheimer's disease, they really think of as deserved punishment. Hostility and anger can erupt, and caregiving may be difficult for such family members to provide. This is a family situation that is at risk for abuse to occur. However, the affected relative's "sin" of commission or omission did not cause the Alzheimer's-type condition.

The family adjustment process can sometimes bring up beliefs about why the loved one has developed Alzheimer's disease. These beliefs, unlike those just described, usually represent family members' attempts to come to terms with this illness.

A history of psychiatric problems does not increase risk.

People who have had psychiatric problems throughout their lives are not necessarily more susceptible to Alzheimer's disease. However, some families may believe that psychiatric illnesses, such as chronic depression, are responsible for later brain disorders. There is virtually no evidence for this contention. One research report suggests that persons with Alzheimer's disease do seem to have a higher incidence of psychiatric episodes, especially depression, which occur much earlier than the onset of the disease's symptoms (Agbayewa 1986).

Psychiatric episodes often are precursors to more obvious symptoms of dementia.

The author of this research suggests that the psychiatric episodes could conceivably represent prodromal stages of the illness. In addition to depression, paranoid disorders were strongly implicated as potential forerunners of the Alzheimer's-type dementia (Agbayewa 1986). This area of research should be continued; however, the reported findings should be viewed cautiously.

Psychiatric symptoms can be manifested during the course of Alzheimer's disease. Delusions, hallucinations, agitation, anxiety, depression, and catastrophic reactions can all occur. Psychiatric manifestations, their intensity and duration can vary from one individual to another. The environment, which includes the family, has some influence.

Sensory impairments contribute to hallucinations and delusions.

Sensory impairments such as existing visual and hearing problems contribute to individual variations. For instance, persons with significant hearing impairment can be more susceptible to auditory hallucinations, even when they do not have Alzheimer's disease. Limitations in reasoning and interpretation of sounds in Alzheimer's create a greater chance of hallucinations, and delusions sometimes develop out of these hallucinations.

Personality factors enter into psychiatric symptoms which accompany Alzheimer's disease. By the time an individual develops this condition, his personality traits are well defined. Enduring characteristics of the person, how he behaves socially, and how he typically responds to situations are indicators of his personality. Suspicious and paranoid types may become more agitated and distrustful when they have Alzheimer's disease. A person who has always been dependent will become more dependent and insecure.

Familiar, well-organized, comfortable environment minimizes coping problems. Environmental factors, including physical arrangement and social and psychological overtones, exert considerable influences on how individuals cope with Alzheimer's disease. The caregiving environment will also determine to a degree the effectiveness and endurance of the caregiver. A familiar, well-organized, and comfortable environment can be supportive of Alzheimer's care. Good lighting during the day and enough lighting at night to help the patient find the bathroom can be helpful. Later, signs can be used to indicate the bathroom door. A poster with important reminders, names, and phone numbers can increase the security of some Alzheimer's patients when the caregiver must be gone for a short while. The house can be secured at night to prevent the patient's wandering outside the home. Additionally, the household can be run in a calm, relaxed manner to reduce unnecessary noise and unsettling distractions.

Social contact is important for both patient and caregiver Complete social isolation is harmful for both the caregiver and the patient. Outside social contact need not be lengthy for the Alzheimer's patient, but some degreee of consistency from friends and other family helps maintain a sense of a social bond. For example, the length of visits can be preset and arranged to include both the patient and the caregiver. When the patient begins to tire and withdraw somewhat from the conversation, the visitor can spend some focused time with the caregiver, satisfying both persons' need for social interaction. At times, those who have Alzheimer's disease are self-conscious about their limitations and may leave the room even when visitors are still there. Both visitors and caregiver should accept the departure without protest; the patient should not be forced to stay. Additionally, caregivers need to reassure the affected relatives that they are loved and accepted in spite of the disease.

Psychological environment

The psychological environment should be encouraging and supportive. A calm atmosphere has a more relaxing effect on both the patient and the caregiver. Of course, some stimulation and activity must be preserved according to the capabilities of the person receiving the care. Too many demends may create more restlessness and agitation. The affected relative should no longer be held accountable for many of his mistakes and errors in judgment. The caregivers' insistent correction can result in more reactive responses from the patient. Any opportunity to support the shrinking self-esteem of the Alzheimer's patient must be acted upon. Meaningful rewards are important, even for helping with the smallest of tasks.

In this book, a great deal of emphasis is placed on the beliefs of family members concerning the changed behavior of their affected relative. When families can understand more of their relative's behavior from the perspective of brain impairment, they can relate more successfully to that behavior. Their responses can be more sensitive without as much anger and frustration. Uninformed and overburdened caregivers have attributed intricate intellectual plans to loved ones, believing that the brain-impaired person consciously followed these plans to get what he wanted or to repay the caregiver for some supposed insult. It is questionable whether an Alzheimer's patient can respond in such a premeditated manner. It is more likely he is reacting to something in the environment or to his own misinterpretations.

Isolation has a profound effect on elderly persons living alone.

From our community work in geriatric mental health, we have seen the profound effects isolation can have on some elderly who live alone. They are referred to us for treatment when they seem to be a danger to themselves or seem unable to provide for their most basic needs. Most often family or neighbors notice unusual or frightening behavior and call us for help. When we go to the home to check out these reports, we often find the house in disarray, cans of open food on the cabinets, decomposing items in the refrigerator, and unopened take-out lunches from the senior center on the counter. Sometimes we find the person just lying on the floor in a heap. In some instances, these people may be defensive when they see us, but often they try to be cordial and friendly. They are bewildered by troubles they cannot seem to handle on their own, but they are frightened to allow strangers to help them (a reasonable response even if the strangers are part of a geriatric mental health team).

In these kind of cases, symptoms of dementia are often present. Many of these persons will eventually be diagnosed as having Alzheimer's disease. Occasionally, reversible medical conditions or pseudodementia are found to be responsible for the functional impairments.

Hearing and visual impairments contribute to isolation.

Hearing and visual impairments often contribute to isolation in the elderly. Sensory and social deprivation are known to have significant impact on a person's functioning, and in the elderly individual with dementia, they suggest that psychosocial factors play a role in precipitating delusions and hallucinations. Interestingly, the hallucinations and delusions in this context may be attempts at creating stimulation in a world that has shrunk to the parameters of a couple of rooms. The isolated person with dementia is stuck between the insecurity of memory problems and the fear of other people taking over his life.

Reaction to nursing home placement is influenced by benefits perceived in the move.

Eventually the Alzheimer's patient may have to be placed in a nursing home or other 24-hour facility. Placing a family member in a nursing home is a difficult decision for families involved in Alzheimer's care. However, relocation effects on the patient are influenced by the person's perception of loss of control along with other aspects of the move.

Thus it is how the living situation changes, not the change itself that is important. If the relocation improves the person's living situation, its effects will not be detrimental. For example, persons make a better adjustment to a nursing home relocation if they perceive the care as better, have easier accessibility to their physician, have meaningful things to do, and have the opportunity to make friends.

The factors above increase security and, consequently, the person's sense of control because there is more positively defined predictability in his life. However, of the factors that indicate quality, one is more significant than all the others: the extent of social support the person perceives himself to receive. It is the emotional response induced by the change, not the change itself, that is vital (Henry 1986).

More advanced Alzheimer's patients do not have the intellectual capacity necessary to adjust to a new environment without considerable assistance. However, they may relate most often—at a basic emotional level—to what is happening to and around them, as their ability to reason and make intellectual judgments fades.

These observations have applications to caregiving even when there is no relocation in the immediate future. A strong sense of social support is critical to persons with Alzheimer's disease whether they are living in nursing homes or in their own homes. Deprived environments can precipitate "excessive disability" and "learned helplessness," while supportive and stimulating environments encourage individuals to maintain more control of their lives and be a little more involved in the world outside of themselves.

Uncertainty and risk   Not knowing what causes Alzheimer's is a psychosocial factor of the disease which often has negative effects on dementia patients and their caregivers. Family history has been a known risk factor; persons who have a first-degree relative with Alzheimer's may have a fourfold increase in risk for getting the disease (Weiner and Gray 1996). Other risk factors have been identified: aging (the older we get, the greater the chance we will develop the disease), head injury associated with hospitalization or loss of consciousness, history of severe depression, history of Parkinson's disease in a first-degree relative, and possibly advanced maternal age (Katzman 1996). Educational level is a possible risk factor. Lower educational level may increase the risk; more years of formal education may delay or decrease the chance of developing Alzheimer's later in life. Anti-inflammatories and estrogen have been implicated as having a role in reducing risk.

A recent study has drawn the tentative conclusion that Japanese-American men who have moved from Japan to Hawaii are more susceptible to developing Alzheimer's disease (White 1996). This finding points to the fact that culture and environment may carry risk factors. No known evidence supports one race being more or less vulnerable to the disease on that basis alone. Women may have a higher risk, but this may be a result of their living longer than men. There are no diet or nutritional factors that are known to play a role in developing Alzheimer's and that have been supported by research.

Most negative and positive risk factors are beyond our control. There is one notable exception: educational level attained. It appears that there is some degree of truth to the old idea that we will lose our mental capacity if we fail to use it and learn. Learning at any age is generative or regenerative from a neurobiological perspective.

Community resources need to be increased.
For this long moment in time, while we wait for a cure or treatment, we must use what we know to make the lives of individuals with Alzheimer's disease as well as the family caregivers safer and more meaningful. Other approaches to long-term care must be developed. Many communities are still lacking the resources to support Alzheimer's services, such as day and respite care. Families often feel less helpless in dealing with this illness if they are involved in support groups. Political action has already paid off for Alzheimer's research, but more research and care options are needed. Families can work with their own legislators or city officials to gather more support for funding vital services. Area Agencies on Aging can help develop options.

Families must not be afraid to seek available help.
Just doing something about the situation often counteracts feelings of helplessness and hopelessness. Families must be willing to seek help when they need it, particularly when help is available. Certainly Alzheimer's disease can be described in tragic terms, but there are other tragedies which can often be prevented. One example is the suffering that families experience when they are unwilling to seek help that is available. Another example is the suffering added to the lives of persons experiencing or dealing with Alzheimer's disease by insensitive professionals who project their own hopelessness into the lives of those they are charged with helping. Such needless pain can and must be prevented.

5

SIX COMMON MYTHS
ABOUT ALZHEIMER'S

Families hold misconceptions. Many misconceptions exist about the nature of Alzheimer's disease. Lacking adequate information about the disease, families commonly hold mistaken notions about the disease itself, old age, and their own role in caring for the person with Alzheimer's. In addition, they may harbor unnecessary fears about the likelihood that they will inherit the disease from their relative.

Because our beliefs are the basis for our actions, it is important that families have an accurate understanding of Alzheimer's and its significance. The following are some of the most common myths about Alzheimer's, followed by a correct assessment of the pertinent issues.

Myth 1: Alzheimer's Symptoms Are a Normal Sign of Old Age

Alzheimer's should not be confused with the aging process. Some of the early symptoms of Alzheimer's, such as forgetfulness, do correspond to our common notions of aging; but Alzheimer's is a disease and should not be confused with the aging process. This becomes clear as the disease progresses, and the victim's deterioration becomes more dramatic.

Old-age forgetfulness is benign. In terms of memory loss, for example, it is true that a degree of increased forgetfulness commonly accompanies aging. Older persons may find it more difficult to recall the details of past events. However, the memory loss caused by Alzheimer's is far more severe and progressive in nature. Eventually the disease destroys not just the memory of details but all memory of the event itself. The person in time will forget not only the events of the past but what she did that morning, who her spouse is, where she lives, even her own name. These are not the normal consequences of aging.

Myth 2: Senility Is the Usual Cause of Problems in Old Age

Senility obscures real illnesses and problems of aging. Senility is a blanket term that has long been used to cover a wide-ranging variety of symptoms. In this sense it is a damaging notion and a term to be avoided. An assumed diagnosis of senility obscures the real problem at hand and increases the difficulty of getting correct treatment for the older person's condition or impairment. The older person may suffer along assuming her condition is irreversible, when treatment may in fact be readily available. In addition, the myth of senility reinforces the negative and mistaken belief that all persons must become helpless and useless with age.

Common hearing and visual problems produce misleading views of older persons. If an older person has difficulty relating to others or conducting her affairs, many problems other than senility or Alzheimer's disease may be the source. For example, the person may suffer from impaired hearing or vision. Her failure to clearly follow a conversation or respond to something in the environment may make it seem that her thought processes are impaired, when actually she has simply not seen or heard what happened. Additionally, the impaired person may begin to avoid situations where her problem is most apparent or troublesome. A person who is hard of hearing may avoid crowds, while a person with poor sight may become confused in social situations because everyone's face looks the same. Often older persons are unwilling to admit these impairments, which can add to confusion about the source of their problems.

Medical problems produce emotional and behavioral changes labeled as senility.

Medical conditions also may be at the root of the older person's problems. Congestive heart failure may cause weakness, fatigue, mental confusion, forgetfulness, and other symptoms mistaken for senility. Hyperthyroidism may cause apathy, depression, lethargy, impaired memory, and slow responses in the elderly. Hypothyroidism has similar symptoms in the elderly, with weakness and fatigue a little more prominent. Both of these illnesses have a slow, progressive onset similar to that of Alzheimer's disease. Persons suffering from these problems should receive a full medical evaluation, and family members should not just assume that the problem is old age.

Other conditions that may be confused with Alzheimer's include B-12 deficiencies, pernicious anemia, electrolyte imbalances, normal pressure hydrocephalus, hypoglycemia, and a range of infections. Infections of the urinary system, for example, may cause confusion, apathy, and inattentiveness before other symptoms are apparent. It is therefore essential that experienced medical personnel rule out all other possible causes for the older person's problems before arriving at a diagnosis of Alzheimer's.

Medications create Alzheimer's-type symptoms.

Often medication prescribed for a medical condition can cause side effects similar to Alzheimer's symptoms, such as confusion, forgetfulness, tremors, and slower responses. This can be a particular problem when the older person is taking several medications at one time to treat different conditions. If problems are apparent, they should be brought promptly to the attention of the doctor or doctors involved. When a number of doctors and pharmacies are involved with different medications, there is a greater chance that medication-related problems will develop. It is therefore extremely important to provide all professionals involved with an up-to-date regimen of medications.

Depression is often mistaken for senility.

Psychological problems such as depression often are passed off as senility as well. It is common for older persons to experience some depression as they face the loss of health, friends, spouse, home, as well as their own death. Such major life changes late in life may lead to mental conditions requiring a psychiatrist's care, such as severe depression, anxiety, or paranoia. The person may not seem "crazy," but fear and insecurity in the face of real losses or perceived threats may be interfering with her ability to effectively cope with life.

Depression accentuates other difficulties. Depression can in turn lead to complaints about memory problems. The person may see even minor memory lapses as evidence that she is becoming senile. In fact, however, she may simply be suffering from lapses in attention and concentration caused by the depression. One difference between the symptoms of depression and those of Alzheimer's is that, while the depressed person may not recognize her depression, she will rarely deny the resulting problems. Alzheimer's victims, on the other hand, tend to deny all evidence of the disease.

A belief in senility stops people from seeking help. The myth of senility and the lack of dignity associated with it often prevent older persons from seeking treatment for conditions that are in fact reversible. Family members should encourage older persons to seek medical treatment for the problems they encounter and should not let them assume that senility is a necessary consequence of old age.

Myth 3:   Nothing Can Be Done for the Alzheimer's Victim

Proper care is important in the management of the illness. It is true that at present we have no cure for Alzheimer's disease. The disease is progressive and leads ultimately to death. However, there is much that can be done to make the victim's last months or years more meaningful, pleasant, and comfortable.

Medical care Alzheimer's patients benefit from both proper medical care and informed behavior management. Thus the family should involve health professionals in their victim's care as early as possible, and they should continue to seek professional opinions throughout the disease.

Psychiatric care

Psychiatrists and other mental health professionals can successfully treat the depression or other psychological symptoms that frequently develop. Doctors and nutritionists can provide help with meal preparation, special diets, and nutritional supplements as the person's appetite and eating abilities deteriorate. Careful attention to the use of medications will prevent unnecessary and prolonged side effects.

Other medical problems coexist.

Treatment of coexisting medical problems is also very important. It should not be assumed that all of the person's physical and mental symptoms are caused by the disease. Persons with Alzheimer's are especially vulnerable to the common viruses, colds, and infections that affect us all, including pneumonia, and these conditions should receive prompt medical attention.

Myth 4: Alzheimer's Is Strictly a Mental Illness

Psychiatric symptoms

Many of the changes initially observed in the Alzheimer's patient seem to be personality disorders or other psychological problems. Furthermore, because Alzheimer's disease primarily affects the brain, it is in a sense a "mental" illness. However, Alzheimer's disease is a degenerative medical condition and not a psychiatric disorder.

Psychiatric symptoms are a significant part of the illness. As the brain gradually loses its capacity to perform normal functions we take for granted, the individual becomes increasingly insecure and unable to relate to her daily world. In time her personality is completely altered, and she truly becomes a "different person" than the loved one we have always known.

Insurance views the illness as psychiatric.

Because society's recognition of the medical nature of the disease is fairly recent, however, Alzheimer's may be regarded at times as a psychiatric condition. Persons financially dependent on insurance or Medicaid programs, for example, may find that they do not meet the "medical" requirements that make them eligible for long-term care. It is to be hoped that these requirements and attitudes will change as the understanding of Alzheimer's becomes more widespread.

Diagnostic findings of good health are misleading.

The impression that Alzheimer's is a mental illness may be supported when a diagnosis of general "good health" is coupled with a diagnosis of Alzheimer's disease. What medical professionals mean by such a diagnosis, however, is that no other medical problems have been found, or other conditions are so successfully controlled that the individual is in otherwise satisfactory health.

Myth 5:   Only the Family Should Care for the Alzheimer's Victim

Family care is supportive and necessary.

In most cases, it is certainly best if the affected person can stay at home with her spouse or family as long as possible. The love and regular interaction a family can provide usually helps the person retain her abilities longer and helps ease her difficult adjustment to the disease.

Other resources make a big difference.

However, not all spouses or children have the resources to care properly for their loved one. Even those who do have the resources eventually may have to call upon outside care when the disease reaches its later stages and caregiving becomes an utterly exhausting experience.

Caregivers should be careful about overinvolvement. Overinvolvement, or the feeling that the caregiver must do everything herself, is a common reaction to the disease. Often it represents a stage in the family member's adjustment to the disease (see Chapter 8). The caregiver imagines that she can hold back the disease by doing everything herself, and her grief leads her to become extremely protective of the victim. She may also feel reluctant to seek outside help because of shame and the stigmas associated with mental conditions.

Primary caregivers must accept help. However, the family, and in particular the primary caregiver, must learn to accept help. The burden of caring for an Alzheimer's patient can otherwise cause serious problems for the caregiver and alienate her from friends and family who want to share the caregiving role. The caregiver should not hesitate to call upon community resources as well, such as those discussed in detail in Chapter 13. Without these resources, the burden of care can be overwhelming.

Myth 6: All Relatives of Alzheimer's Victims Are Likely to Inherit the Disease

Facts of genetic risk It is common for relatives of Alzheimer's disease victims to be concerned that they may have a genetic predisposition toward the disease. When the first edition of this book was published in 1988, a few families in which early-onset Alzheimer's (before age 65, usually starting in the forties or fifties) was documented were known to have a pattern of inheritance known as autosomal-dominant. If one parent had a defective gene, each child had a 50 percent chance of inheriting the gene. These persons would not necessarily develop the disease at an early age—or ever develop it. For the individuals at risk in this family, waiting determined whether or not they developed the disease.

**Familial
Alzheimer's
disease**
The family knew, however, that some members would eventually develop the disease, because members of other generations were known to have had it. Because the disease developed with some degree of frequency in these families, it is called familial Alzheimer's disease. From one generation to the next, the disease continued to appear in yet another family member. Early-onset Alzheimer's cases are likely to represent this form of the disease. It may develop in some persons when they are in their early thirties.

**Early-onset
genetics**
These early-onset forms of familial Alzheimer's disease with autosomal-dominant inheritance are rare. They are associated with mutations of genes on three different chromosomes: 1, 14, and 21. Members of these families may have a basis for concern about developing Alzheimer's. Family history of known or suspected Alzheimer's must be documented. It may not be easy, or even possible in some family histories, to track and document instances of Alzheimer's disease. Not all early-onset familial cases can be explained by genetic mutations. It is likely there are still other genes to be identified for this form of the disease. Since other early-onset cases appear to be more sporadic, interaction between both genetic and non-genetic factors may be present.

**Late-onset
genetics**
For late-onset (age 65 and older) Alzheimer's disease, it has been more difficult to establish the role of genetic inheritance. Experts estimate that roughly 98 percent of Alzheimer's patients develop the late-onset kind of Alzheimer's (Stephenson, 1997). Some late-onset familial and sporadic forms of the disease have been linked to the apoE gene mutation on chromosome 19. There are three forms, or alleles, of this gene: E2, E3, and E4. ApoE4 is found in about 40 percent of late-onset Alzheimer's disease patients, and is the form of apoE that increases a person's susceptibility to the disease. Persons with familial and sporadic forms of Alzheimer's disease have this gene, and the number (having one or two E4 genes) has an influ-

ence on how great one's risk is for the disease, and at what age it develops.

Newer evidence suggests that apoE4 may be a risk factor only for patients who develop Alzheimer's before age 70, and because more than 90 percent of Alzheimer's cases occur in persons older than 70, there is very good reason to continue the search for other genetic evidence linked to the most common form of the disease.

Genetic tests   The identification of the apoE gene and its association with Alzheimer's has created interest in the use of a genetic screening test that might identify or predict risk for Alzheimer's. ApoE is not a consistent biological marker for the disease; screening for it would miss some persons with Alzheimer's and falsely identify others. For this reason a public policy statement concerning genetic testing was developed at a conference sponsored by the National Institute on Aging and Alzheimer's Association in October 1995. ApoE testing is appropriate for use in research settings that incorporate much broader protocols for diagnostic purposes and that consider apoE testing only when persons are concerned about symptoms suggesting Alzheimer's disease. Genetic counseling is recommended for research volunteers and their families so that they can learn about the genetics of the disease, the tests being used, and the meaning of the results.

For families who do face the possibility of an inherited form of Alzheimer's, involvement with research centers provides the chance for information, care, and support. These families can see that, although the numbers may be small, other families are also dealing with the ongoing plague Alzheimer's unleashes on them. Family members who collaborate with researchers in a meaningful way and feel they are making a contribution to this area of research may gain a greater sense of mastery over this part of their lives, which seems beyond control.

6

COPING: A STEP-BY-STEP GUIDE TO THE CAREGIVER'S EXPERIENCE

A hypothetical case history Eleanor is becoming increasingly concerned about her husband Bill. He has made some errors in his checkbook, which are uncharacteristic, and twice recently he has gotten lost driving in unfamiliar parts of town. Yet when she brings her concerns up, he becomes angry and denies everything. At first, she associated these problems with getting old. Bill does have early cataracts and does not see well. But now he is becoming suspicious of her and the neighbors. Recently she was shocked when he confronted a neighbor about stealing tools out of the garage. He had never done anything like that before.

During the last few years, Eleanor has heard a great deal about Alzheimer's disease. She is afraid that something like that might be happening to Bill. Her husband is slowly changing, and she feels a growing pressure to do something. But what? Should she talk to the family doctor or a psychiatrist? It has always been difficult to get Bill to see a doctor, and Bill keeps insisting that he has no problems. Bill's behavior is becoming embarrassing to Eleanor, which makes her reluctant to do things with her friends. She does not know how to tell the children about her fears, and since they both live out of state, they have not seen for themselves what is happening to their father. Whenever Eleanor thinks about the changes in Bill, she feels alone and afraid.

Responding to Alzheimer's symptoms is difficult. Eleanor's predicament is typical of the difficult situation in which relatives of persons in the early stages of Alzheimer's often find themselves. They feel certain that something is very wrong, but they do not know what they should do to help. Never having experienced anything like this before and afraid that the problem may be more serious than they can bear, they feel at a loss to identify the first step.

Knowing what lies ahead helps. This chapter seeks to alleviate the confusion and anxiety that caregivers experience by offering a step-by-step guide to the process of coping with Alzheimer's disease. It outlines the steps that caregivers will need to take and offers helpful, practical advice for what to do at each stage. By clearly identifying the disease process and the challenges that lie ahead for the caregiver, the information in this chapter aims to relieve the anxiety caregivers feel in facing an unknown threat. The following are the steps discussed in depth in this chapter.

1. Noticing initial symptoms
2. Confirming suspicions
3. Seeking information
4. Taking action
5. Weighing findings
6. Identifying resources
7. Planning care
8. Managing caregiver stress

1. Noticing Initial Symptoms

All illnesses have symptoms. If the problem is a physical one, the symptoms are likely to be familiar physical complaints such as fever, headache, nausea, fatigue, and specific areas of pain. The signs of mental illness can be more difficult to identify, yet symptoms are still present. Persons suffering from depression, for example, may not recognize that they are depressed, yet they often report symptoms. Similarly, persons with Alzheimer's may experience symptoms but fail to attribute them to a brain condition.

Early symptoms may not clearly suggest Alzheimer's disease. With Alzheimer's, symptoms observed early in the illness are likely to be behavioral or emotional, and the person's distress is usually psychological. He probably will not associate his initial problems with an intellectual function such as memory or suspect that a serious illness is the cause. Though a spouse or other relative may observe slight changes in the person's normal behavior, it is difficult to take these changes seriously at first.

Denial of symptoms is common. The affected person may feel that acknowledging his difficulties would create unnecessary worries for his family or place his job in jeopardy. He may feel that he can overcome these problems if he tries harder.

Often, when he discovers that he can do little about his memory problems, he will become noticeably anxious, frustrated, and irritable with the possibility of depression developing. It is common for the affected person to point out memory lapses of other family members to distract attention from his own growing difficulties.

Symptoms become harder to ignore. However, the person's memory problems, as well as his emotional and behavioral reactions, will begin eventually to create genuine concern among family members. They will begin to wonder if perhaps the changes and deficiencies they are noticing might be symptoms of something larger.

2. Confirming Suspicions

Families must seek professional help. Families usually discuss early concerns with other family and friends first. As initial doubts become more persistent, they generally feel a need to share their concerns with a health professional who can positively confirm or deny their suspicions.

It is important to consult a health professional as soon as possible, for a preliminary medical consultation will

- Clarify the seriousness of the problems
- Verify the need for action
- Ensure prompt treatment if the condition is not in fact Alzheimer's.

A professional provides both medical information and emotional support.

Often, it is difficult to get the person to agree to see a doctor, and many families are reluctant to take a relative to a health professional without consent. When this problem arises, the family may wish to consult a doctor or a mental health professional on their own. Contact with a professional can

- Give initial feedback on whether the symptoms described sound like those associated with Alzheimer's
- Suggest where to go for a comprehensive evaluation of the relative's condition, and explain the costs and time involved
- Address the fears, doubts, and confusion of family members about what needs to be done. (This area alone justifies contact with a professional familiar with Alzheimer's disease.)

If the family can provide the professional with a list of problems and examples of symptoms observed, this will help the professional make a determination of a person's condition.

Use of Behavior Profile

Included in the appendix is a "Behavior Profile" which is a comprehensive listing of difficulties ranging from orientation to behavior problems. This scale is helpful for families in documenting problems and their frequency. The profile also provides the caregiver with an opportunity to determine how stressful he finds a particular behavior. It will be useful later in the illness to determine the amount of assistance a person requires and specific behaviors that require more intervention and supportive counseling to relieve the stress surrounding such behaviors.

Families should establish a clear history of symptoms.

The history of symptoms and problems is extremely important in making an accurate diagnosis. Families should note how long they have observed various symptoms in their relative. A number of illnesses such as depression and strokes without motor impairment have symptoms that are very similar to those characteristic of Alzheimer's disease. A good history of such symptoms will reflect whether they developed suddenly or over an extended period. Such information becomes significant in the evaluation of this illness.

3. Seeking Information

Community resources provide information and support.

In addition to consulting a family doctor, neurologist, psychiatrist, or other mental health professional, the family may wish to seek information on Alzheimer's disease from an Alzheimer's Family Support Group or an Alzheimer's Resource Center. Family support meetings can put a family in touch with vital local resources as well as with professionals who are experienced in diagnosing Alzheimer's disease.

4. Taking Action

A full evaluation involves several health professionals.

An appointment with the family physician may be the starting point for the evaluative process, with basic tests ordered. Often the physician may refer his patient to another professional, such as a neurologist, psychiatrist, or a mental health center for evaluation.

Since the family has decided to act, they want results and some answers. What will help? What can be done to manage the situation even though no cure exists? The family probably expects a medication to manage symptoms. The family's need for information accelerates after the implications of the diagnosis are recognized.

Seeking a second opinion may be necessary.   If a physician gives the diagnosis of Alzheimer's after minimal testing, the family may experience a letdown that can create distrust, lack of confidence in the physician, and real dissatisfaction. A similar situation exists when incorrect diagnosis of senility or hardening of the arteries is given to informed family members who are keenly aware of their loved one's extreme degree of impairment. Not all doctors are experts in diagnosing and managing the disease, and families should not hesitate to seek a second opinion if they feel dissatisfied with the first diagnosis. If Alzheimer's is suspected, a doctor with a particular expertise in the disease should be consulted—even if this means traveling to another city.

5. Weighing Findings

Families must evaluate the implications of a diagnosis.   After initial diagnostic evaluations have been completed, family members are faced with several tasks including:

a. Questioning the diagnosis and considering the need for a second opinion

b. Understanding the implications of this diagnosis, particularly when confusing, conflicting, or inaccurate information and advice from both professional and nonprofessional sources must be reconciled

c. Reaching a family consensus about what needs to be done now, and in the future, and by whom

d. Deciding whether others should be told about the Alzheimer's condition.

6. Identifying Resources

Alzheimer's as yet cannot be cured. However, some of the related problems can be managed and even treated with medication and proper behavioral management.

Families must realistically assess resources. Before embarking upon a plan of management for the disease and care for the person affected, family members need to realistically assess their personal resources in both emotional and financial terms and examine those offered in the community. Personal resources in this sense are determined by the following factors:

a. The physical health of the most likely primary caregiver

b. The availability of community support and resources

c. The caregiver's living situation and the proximity of other involved family members

d. The family's financial resources and the victim's eligibility for publicly funded services

e. The strength of the caregiver's marital relationship (Can it withstand the stresses of continuous caregiving?)

f. The availability of transportation

g. The availability of family, friends, or paid help to take over care of patient for several hours at least twice a week

h. The availability of persons who fill the role of confidant.

Compensating for changes in one's personal/social supports
Caregivers must realize the support system of friends and family that has helped them in previous times of trouble may not be enough to get them through the stresses of caring for their loved one. Alzheimer's caregiving can last a long time. The family caregiver must assess the potential support available during the caregiving process as realistically as possible and begin to find replacements for the emotional support previously provided by the victim himself.

The caregiver can use the "Personal/Social Support Resources" form in the appendix to assess the degree of support that is currently available. Caregivers must realize that they need support for themselves, too. If the affected family member has been the primary source of support, new resources must be actively sought out.

7. Planning Care

A plan is necessary.
Planning the care of an Alzheimer's victim can seem to be a confusing and perhaps even unnecessary task (especially when the patient is not exhibiting serious management problems). However, as time moves on and the disease progresses, it will become obvious that a plan is necessary.

A home-care planning list is in the Appendix.
To begin the care-planning process, a "Family In-Home Behavior Care List" is included in the appendix. The questions on the list will help a family identify areas in which their relative needs assistance and how much assistance is needed.
Caregivers must begin to prioritize needs, and they must decide who best can deliver the needed help. They must realize that their lives are changed by the disease, and they must change their approaches accordingly.

Problem behavior needs careful consideration. Other approaches to problem-solving should be considered in family care planning.

a. When do problem behaviors occur, and what else is happening when these problems surface? (For example, is the person more difficult and irritable when the television is playing loudly?)

b. What occurs before or after the undesired behavior? Are these events or conditions producing and rewarding the undesired behavior?

c. How frequently does the problem occur? Is it really that big a problem?

d. How severe or dangerous is the problem?

e. Can advance planning reduce opportunities for the problem behavior to occur?

Case example of problem-solving Emma started calling for her husband at night after she had gone to bed. He usually helped her to bed about 10 P.M. and then stayed up a while alone. She usually fell asleep before she awoke in a panic calling for her husband, somewhat confused. Her husband always turned the light off before going into the den for his quiet time. Because she was so afraid, her husband always ran to her rescue, most often holding her and falling asleep with her. Night after night, she became frightened when she awoke in the dark. As a consequence, her husband had very little time to himself.

Emma's husband realized he was reinforcing her behavior—the calls at night increased. He also realized that waking in the dark might be frightening to Emma. To deal with the problem he did several things.

- He spent more intimate time with his wife before she went to sleep
- He left a lamp on in the bedroom while she was asleep

■ When she called for him, he called back to her, reassuring her he was just down the hall in the den. Most of the time Emma went back to sleep, and her husband could continue relaxing alone.

8. Managing Caregiver Stress

Stress from caregiving is not necessarily a result of the Alzheimer's condition.

Too often the stress of caregiving is attributed solely to the condition of the relative with Alzheimer's. As his condition worsens, the stress experienced by the family caregiver increases. This point of view fails to appreciate other aspects of the caregiving situation, which in turn can make it more difficult for the caregiver to cope effectively with the needs of his relative. More contact from friends and relatives provides for the social and emotional support needs that have increased during the caregiver's physical isolation of more solitary care situations. Utilization of available resources is another factor influencing the caregivers perception of stress. Resources can actually allow the caregiver to participate more in the community.

Other factors influence caregiver stress.

The age of the caregiver may influence the degree of stress he experiences. Younger caregivers may have other career and family responsibilities that conflict with full assumption of the caregiving role. The type of role change created by caregiving also influences the degree of stress that will be experienced. For example, female caregivers may resent a return to the caregiver role itself when it had been abandoned for a career after children were grown. Some men, on the other hand, may view the role change associated with a new "provider" role more satisfying. Nurturing his ill spouse offers the male a way to repay his wife for her earlier role in family nurturing.

Caregivers need to help themselves. The stresses of caregiving are not simply the result of the continued deterioration of the relative affected. The well-being of the family caregiver is essential. One of the purposes for an Alzheimer's Family Support Group is to help family members cope successfully with the illness. Counseling also can be sought. Caregivers may prevent some stress by utilizing their personal/social support resources.

Caregivers can do much to help themselves. They should explore community services, and they must recognize their limitations, especially during a long period of intense care. Without outside support, caregivers can develop stress-induced illnesses such as depression and anxiety (see Chapter 3 on Depression and Alzheimer's). Medical problems such as hypertension, diabetes, and heart conditions may worsen because of prolonged stress and poorer self-care.

A stress test is included in the appendix. The "Care Management Stress" scale included in the appendix can help families identify specific stress areas. The areas include stress created by family expectations, isolation, problem behaviors, an uncertain future, and the inherent burden of day-to-day care. In responding to the questions, the caregiver should note the frequency of each response and his emotional response to each statement and make care decisions accordingly.

A stress scale for institutional caregivers is a good preventive tool. Staff of nursing homes and other institutionals also can experience stress as they see the consequences of the illness daily. A "Staff Stress Measure" is included in the appendix. Training and other educational opportunities can help staff understand Alzheimer's, deal with behavior effectively and compassionately, and manage the stress associated with such care.

Both the "Care Management Stress" scale and the "Staff Stress Measure" can be scored. The higher the score, the higher is the potential for stress. More importantly, caregivers can identify particularly stressful areas and give them more attention.

Managing stress is an ongoing activity.

Managing stress is an ongoing activity. Different features of the patient's progressive condition precipitate new problems and stressors. For example, the first time the Alzheimer's patient fails to recognize his spouse may be so shocking that the caregiver's adjustment is set back considerably.

Stress is likely to grow.

As the patient's condition worsens, the stress felt by the caregiver is likely to grow. He should therefore be willing to continuously reassess the possibility of seeking outside help in some form. These resources range from day or respite care to psychiatric hospitalization or nursing home admission. Outpatient mental health services also should be considered as the burdens placed on the caregiver mount.

Look for positive experiences in caregiving.

There are many ways to change the negatives of this illness into some unexpected positives. Opportunities actually surface from the most unexpected situations, which may lead to new experiences or back to old experiences and activities that seemed to have been lost.

Some examples of the positive aspects of caregiving

Thomas became the caregiver for his wife about six months ago. He had been doing the cooking and washing. Then his wife required help with bathing and dressing as well. His "hands-on" care began to increase.

A chance to return years of loving care

After years of working hard while his wife Janet reared their six children (and some would say their seven grandchildren), Thomas saw that he had the chance to give back to Janet all the love and care she had so willing given to her entire family.

A chance to gain unexpected support
Johnnie was almost devastated when she first learned that her husband Ted had Alzheimer's disease. Months later, she became involved in a local Alzheimer's Family Support Group. Over the next few months, she came to know a number of other people in situations like hers. They became close friends and confidantes— something she never thought she would have. For two years she benefitted from their support and concern, and they from hers. When Ted died, these friends stood by her along with her family.

FEELINGS

I've had my wounds
and I'm not sure
anyone knows how to heal them.

The doctors and my friends,
family and others
tell me—

"You've lost so much,
you've nursed your loved one
through a baffling disease—

"You've been ignored
drawn taut—
suffered and cried.

"Now that he
is in a nursing home
and you have help
in caring for him,
you are now free
to live your own life.

"Get out and go—
join clubs—be with people—
develop some hobbies—
travel a bit."

I'm trying—I'm trying—
I know they love me—
in many ways, they're right—

But there are times
when I feel like
crawling into a corner
like a sick cat
and just licking my wounds—

Maybe, maybe—for just a time
there's not much wrong with that.

Maude S. Newton

7

UNDERSTANDING BEHAVIORAL CHANGES

Over an indefinite period of time, Alzheimer's disease destroys many of the brain's billions of nerve cells. Another part of this process disrupts the brain's capacity to produce specialized chemicals that allow nerve cells to communicate information to each other. In the healthy brain, this unique system of nerve cells and their specialized chemical messengers enables us to think and reason, remember and be conscious of our experiences, feel and express emotion, learn and achieve goals, and relate these experiences to one another. Because of our brain, we are able to make adaptive changes in how or where we live.

From the moment a child is born, his development is carefully observed. His smiles suggest he is happy and willing to interact positively with his new world. The first steps or first words are hallmarks of development. We expect the child to grow and develop "normally," to learn and have knowledge. This knowledge, and his use of it, is a part of his identity. Memory allows him to store and retrieve this knowledge as it is needed. Sometimes he is more conscious of what he does than the way his thoughts influence his actions.

Later in his life, he will be asked a question, and if unable to answer it he will say, "Nothing comes to mind." All of us have had this experience many times. We can also recall those times we were under pressure to respond quickly to questions raised in a demanding situation. Much to our dismay we remember thinking how our minds went blank. Situations like this are frustrating.

We suffer greater frustration when we realize it is a little harder to learn or remember something than it used to be. We may experience situations that exceed our ability to adapt them. Despite the extreme stress or health problems we may be experiencing, we conclude our minds are not what they used to be. And if we continue to have experiences like these we may translate our frustrations into a belief that imparts greater doubts and concerns. "I'm not what I used to be" or "I'm just not myself anymore." Something unique and treasured about us is threatened—the special relationship between our minds and who we are.

Early Threats to Who We Are

Alzheimer's disease directly affects the way the mind works. Family members become aware of difficulties with memory or changes in behavior long before they discover that these differences represent the beginnings of a disease process. It is normal for families to conclude that dramatic behavioral changes must have something to do with the personality or emotional state of their loved one. For whatever reason, that person's "uniqueness" has changed. That uniqueness is what makes one person different from another. The idea that individuals we know intimately essentially remain the same is important to our relationship. This uniformity persists regardless of age or other factors. Our uniqueness as individuals is more likely to be attributed to our personalities than to our minds. While Alzheimer's disease strips away the memories, behaviors, and abilities held in the mind, its assault on one's personality is not so complete.

Glimmers of the person The personality of your loved one will change, but it happens slowly. As caregiver, you have the chance to observe and relate to many parts of the person that remain unchanged. Even in the more advanced stages of Alzheimer's disease, there will be "glimmers" of the person that was and still is. These glimmers of the person may be sufficient to stimulate other memories; ways he or she was unique, and experiences you shared. These tenuous aspects of your loved one's personality and mind may help sustain you through the caregiving—even through the massive losses you must witness—because there is still evidence of the old self.

The Impact of Losses on Relating

Understanding the relationship between the brain and behavior can help caregivers respond more reasonably to the behavioral changes in their loved one, but not at the expense of their appreciation of what is unique about the person and his or her history. Patterns of behavior and personality characteristics that existed before this disease began to influence his or her involvement with the world may continue. Their expression may not be as appropriate (Shomaker 1987), or they may be more irritating than they used to be. They are not immediately erased.

Threats to relationships
Over time Alzheimer's disease distinctly changes our relationship with the person who has developed this disease. Our personal loss is manifested in the series of losses we witness as our loved ones lose the ability to reason, think, remember, and behave in ways that were uniquely "their ways." Watching them behave differently, with the ability to do less and less for themselves, represents moments of grief for us and for them. In these moments, we realize we are not only losing the person, we are losing the relationship we had with this one we loved. This may be one reason it is so difficult for caregivers to deal with the behavioral changes associated with this disease.

New and unexpected demands to change
As loved ones become less and less like themselves, and act in unusual and unexpected ways, caregivers are confronted by the growing awareness they are on unfamiliar ground. They found their way through uncharted territory before, for instance, when they were first left alone by their mothers at school, had their first date, got married, raised their first child, or started their first job. These experiences were anticipated. They had not occurred without warning. There had been opportunities to prepare for these experiences through education and learning. Caregiver's have no preparation for the changes they experience.

Few family members who become caregivers are experienced in caring for persons who are affected by a progressive form of brain disease like Alzheimer's. As they enter the process of providing care, it is much easier to relate to their loved ones as they always have rather than view their thoughts, behaviors, and moods as the result of brain impairment. It is difficult at first to appreciate how this applies to the caregiver situation and the problems with which caregivers must contend. How much of what happens is related to disease? How much is related to personality, relationships, or the environment?

Attempts to Understand Behavior

People need to understand "why" things happen. They want to know what causes problems so they can solve or prevent them. If your husband has always been reasonably responsive to doing the things you ask him to do, then this expectation does not immediately change just because he has Alzheimer's disease. If you ask him to get dressed and find he is still sitting on the bed fifteen minutes later, you are inclined to think he is deliberately being uncooperative. If he says he can't dress himself, you may believe he is not trying hard enough. On the other hand, you might believe the problem has something to do with you, or what you have done. Maybe grandchildren are visiting and their excitement while they play is simply too much for your husband to handle.

Who is to blame
Some family caregivers have a tendency to blame the loved one for the agitation, uncooperativeness, and other behavioral problems that make it more difficult to care compassionately. Others blame themselves for the difficulties being experienced. In either case, caregivers occasionally feel frustration, anger, guilt, or hopelessness in caring for their afflicted relatives. But keep in mind that caregivers are attempting to relate to their love one as though he were still the capable person he was before the effects of a disease began to undermine his ability to function without help.

Revising Your Expectations

If there is a specific problem in a caregiver relationship, several approaches to solving the problem naturally occur to us. First, we might expect the other person involved to change. We don't usually like to change ourselves. However, if it seems easier to own up to the problem than argue with the other person, we are more likely to agree to change. Sometimes it seems best to change what initially appeared to cause the problem rather than get the other person involved to act differently. For example, if we can't agree on what program to watch on television, we might just turn off the television. Other times, it's just easier to overlook the problem and attempt to do something else.

Changing beliefs about behavior   Alzheimer's caregivers will benefit if they revise the ways they think about problems and what causes them. Blaming the problems, either on the person affected by the disease, or on yourself is not likely to lead to a solution to the problem. It will simply intensify the unpleasant feelings associated with the situation. As caregivers, you must be able to see how the behavior of a loved one is influenced by your expectations. Do you expect too much or too little? Will you treat the person differently if you expect less of her? If you expect too much will she always get upset?

Adults not children   Caring for an adult who had been fully capable, and who is now becoming progressively more dependent, is "not" the same as caring for a dependent child who is becoming more capable and independent. It is reasonable to expect a child to change her behavior, whether it requires learning a new skill or simply choosing to behave in a more socially appropriate manner. As parents, we consider the child before expecting her to do something. Is she ready to handle this particular task or situation? What is deemed appropriate is measured by where the child is in her development.

Caring for adults with Alzheimer's disease requires caregivers to maintain a similar developmental point of view, but reverse the direction of their expectations. What these adults are capable of doing becomes a matter of what abilities still remain. Appropriate behavior must be defined by standards that acknowledge the effects of progressive damage to the brain. Since there is fluctuation in abilities and the degree of impairments, caregivers must be flexible enough to change expectations from one day to the next. Beliefs appropriate for Alzheimer's care must reflect these differences. The victims of this disease become less and less able to be responsible for their behavior. How well they act and what they are able to do depends in part on the success caregivers have in predicting what their loved one is capable of doing at different times, on different tasks, and in different environments.

Problems and the disease

Years ago it seemed helpful to advise caregivers to attribute problems to the disease itself, and not blame themselves or their loved ones for what happened. If relatives behaved in ways that were uncharacteristic of them, then it was helpful to say that unusual behavior was caused by Alzheimer's disease. Without further explanation, this approach is little different from the idea that since there is no cure, there is nothing one can do. Why try to manage behavior? Anything that happens is the result of a disease that cannot be cured. You can't stop it. Why try? Such a proposition would seem to strengthen one's sense of helplessness and hopelessness.

People have different ways of dealing with the enormity of the disease. For example, recently I was meeting with people who were forming a new support group in a small rural city. One of the persons present had just heard that her father had been diagnosed with Alzheimer's disease. Her mother related to her that the neurologist said her dad had a "little bit" of Alzheimer's. I have no way of knowing what the neurologist actually said, but to this family the idea that a loved one had a "little bit" of Alzheimer's was much easier to acknowledge. One cannot have a little bit of Alzheimer's, although one case may be more advanced than another. Still, having a "touch of it" gives one more time to understand what that means.

Other ways to view problems

Attributing problems to the disease is similar to having a "little bit" of Alzheimer's. It is a point where caregivers begin to understand how to deal with the challenges that lie before them. To offset the impact of the disease's progression, caregivers must have the opportunity to learn other ways to view the problems they encounter. They need to go beyond an understanding that simply explains problems as the result of brain cells being destroyed. They need to feel they have more control over what happens. When they are helping a family member do what he or she used to do, they want to know how to determine if an approach will be successful or if it might cause greater problems.

Questioning Old Beliefs about Behavior

Behavior changes dramatically and unexpectedly with Alzheimer's disease. The ways victims behave seems to have no rhyme or reason. Some changes can indeed be attributed to the fact that Alzheimer's destroys the way the brain works. But what is responsible for the other changes that occur? How can family caregivers feel more assured they are responding to the need of their loved one in the best possible way?

These questions are difficult. Professionals who study behavior—the ways people act and what they do—appreciate the fact we cannot always know "why" people behave as they do. It can be even more difficult to understand why individuals, whose behavior is influenced by brain impairment, act as they do. Why does Mary, who has Alzheimer's disease, explode in rage when her husband repeatedly asks her if she wants to go for a walk? Anthony, whose wife has the disease, is bewildered by her persistent allegations he is having an affair. How could she accuse him of such a thing? Joseph's wife continues to tear clothes out of the dresser drawer each time he puts them back. Is his wife trying to get back at him for something he has done? Do these persons intentionally do these things? Are persons with this disease just naturally mean and belligerent? Does the disease "make" them want to hurt the ones they love?

Intent of behavior   Most of us assume that people "intend" to do whatever it is they do. From the time we were children, we have been taught to be responsible for our actions. We believe we will be held accountable for what we do. If we fail to do what is right or acceptable, it is likely we will be held responsible for our failures. Many of us are harsh judges of ourselves. On other occasions, we make excuses, saying we forgot to do something, or insisting that what happened was not what we intended. Others involved may be reluctant to accept these excuses because they, too, believe behavior is intentional.

It seems we are most convinced something was intentional when it hurts or angers us, makes our day longer, or our lives harder. When we believe the acts or words directed at us were intentional, we personalize them. They anger and hurt us more when they continue, because now it is clear the person has purposely planned what is happening. We are angry and hurt because that was the intended result of a premeditated plan. We can only accept so many "accidents" of behavior.

Stress from intentional beliefs   The idea that behavior is intentional becomes a source of stress in caregiving. This idea is not easy to abandon when family members are caregivers. Even professional caregivers may feel the behavioral problems that confront them are the result of well-planned and purposeful efforts cleverly designed to disrupt the care they are attempting to provide, or simply to get attention. Even in the later stages of the disease, these victims of brain damage are credited with devising grand schemes to sabotage their care or create greater misery for their caregivers.

The following examples may remind caregivers of similar experiences. We will use these examples as we discuss the effects of Alzheimer's disease.

Geneva was getting ready to go to church. Her husband, whom she had just taken from the bathroom and seated so he could watch television, stood up, dropped his pants and promptly soiled himself and the area around him. He had effectively manipulated her into staying with him. She was angry and resentful of the control he still exerted over her life.

Angie, a nurse's aide for 8 months, worked with Alzheimer's patients daily. Today, while she was taking Mr. Knots into a day area, he became agitated and resistant. She had told him she had to hurry so she could take her break. He started yelling "no" loudly and repeatedly, and soon other residents in the area became upset. By the time she and other staff had calmed everyone down it was too late to take her break. When she gave Mr. Knots a resentful glance, he was looking at his feet laughing. What reason had she given him to act this way?

Madge had just finished dressing her husband. He looked nice, and she was excited that her sister would be dropping by shortly. She left her husband sitting in the living room. Even though he did not care for her sister, he had agreed to open the door so Madge could get dressed herself. It wasn't until Madge came out of the bedroom that she saw her husband wasn't where she had left him. The front door was open. Maybe her sister and husband were outside. A quick glance revealed an empty yard. About that time, her sister drove up. Now, she and her sister would spend time together—looking for her husband.

Old beliefs about intent

For couples, relating to one another may have become "second nature" because you are so familiar with each other. You relate to each other as you do because you "know how the other person is." This means that you know what to ask, and how to ask it. You are familiar with what your spouse likes, and what they despise. You know how to get them to do something and when it is useless to try. You know what they can do and if they will support what you do. You even have a reasonable idea of why they do what they do and feel the way they feel about certain things. From this perspective, it is possible to believe behavior is intentional.

Dealing with the behavior changes associated with Alzheimer's disease challenges our beliefs about behavior being intentional and planned. Caregivers must re-examine the relationship they have had with persons now affected by the disease. This involves taking inventory of what you know about their behavior and preferences. It includes recalling how you have dealt with problems in the past that affected your relationship. Some upsetting behaviors may upset you more when you believe they result from personality and the way the person has commonly reacted to past difficulties. Both personality and old styles of coping play a role in the way brain-damaged individuals behave.

Coping styles simpler

Persons experiencing brain impairment tend to retain old coping styles. They are expressed as old habits, or strategies that are simple, straightforward, and more immediate (Mace 1990). John had never liked to stay long at the doctor's office. Now he is even more restless if he must wait very long. Catherine had always been prone to get upset at the smallest thing going wrong. She is now difficult for her husband to manage. Instead of thinking about her husband's request to do something, Dorothy simply says no, or walks away from the situation. When Sarah's daughter asks her about why she didn't eat more, she stated she didn't know.

In an earlier example, Geneva believed her husband had soiled himself to keep her from going to church. If he had often manipulated her in the past, she may have reason to believe this behavior was manipulative. On the other hand, he may not have been aware of his surroundings or his social judgment was faulty. He solved his immediate problem by using the living room floor for a bathroom.

This knowledge about the established patterns of behavior and why it occurs is valuable, but the effects of this disease will begin to disturb these patterns. You will wonder what happened to the predictability you used to take for granted. Combined with a better understanding of how the disease is changing the way loved ones act, this knowledge of the old predictable patterns enables caregivers to learn new ways to interpret the reasons for behavior and modify the ways they interact with their family members. But to be completely open to this view of behavior, it will be helpful to reconsider what is involved in behavior being intentional.

Intentional behavior is directed toward some specific goal or purpose. It may be part of a conscious plan designed to accomplish or achieve something. The brain damage associated with Alzheimer's disease gradually reduces the capacity individuals have for reasoning, planning, and carrying out anything but the most basic demonstrations of goal-directed behavior. These individuals lose sight of the normal consequences of behavior. They can no longer appreciate how their behavior affects others. Because their memory is faulty, they cannot remember what they might have started out doing when you find them standing in the middle of the room looking lost. They are lost in the sense their behavior has no goal or destination.

Victims of beliefs   In the examples given earlier, the caregivers were victims of their own assumptions about intentional behavior. Since their own intentions were clear to them, they assumed their loved ones understood what was expected of them. Everything would go smoothly if everyone did their part. But Geneva's husband didn't use the bathroom when he was supposed to, or in the appropriate way or place. The patient Angie was taking to the day area failed to understand the reason she was in a hurry. He probably sensed she was in a hurry as she rushed him into the confusing social situation represented by the day area. His laughter had no relationship to the frustration she was experiencing. Madge's husband probably simply forgot her sister was coming and wandered off after he opened the door. He was as likely to be in another room of the house as he was wandering down the street.

Admittedly, the intentions of all these caregivers had been disrupted, but not as the result of some willful, premeditated plan made and executed by persons with Alzheimer's disease. Their world of needs, and the behavior produced to satisfy these needs, is much more basic. They may express a desire for something but fail to appreciate that it is impractical, dangerous, or even impossible. They respond to the "small picture," not the "big picture." As a result, they fail to understand the consequences of what they want or do; what they refuse to do or will not accept. They may want to go home to a home that doesn't exist or refuse to allow you to change clothes they have worn for several days. They may do something dangerous, but become angry when you remove them from the dangerous situation. Their behavior in this compressed world will reveal more dramatic examples of poor judgment that seem to have little to do with the reality caregivers perceive.

Behavior con-
trol decreases
Another aspect of our beliefs about behavior affects caregiving, and must be modified so that it can be more realistically applied to the caregiving situation. We believe that people should control their behavior. This expectation requires continual revision as the degree of impairment increases. Ultimately, caregivers must accept the fact loved ones "cannot" control what they do. Their behavior is progressively influenced more by the interactions of others with them, and the environments in which they live.

Feeling the need to urinate will signal the need to use the bathroom, and finding the bathroom will usually not be a problem. Later the person may feel the need to go to the bathroom, but may need reminders or assistance to get to it. The bathroom itself may stimulate its appropriate use for a while. Later reminders or instructions to use the bathroom will be required even when the person has been seated on the commode. Scheduling of routine trips to the bathroom will prevent accidents. Finally the individual will no longer understand what the physical signals of his body mean or recognize what should be done. He cannot control his bladder the way he used to.

In the past, we believed Alzheimer's victims could have tried harder if their level of effort was insufficient for accomplishing something or doing it better. Unfortunately, caregivers still believe that if the victim tries harder he should be able to do things he used to, or at least do better. This belief is fostered by the fact that behavior fluctuates in Alzheimer's victims. One moment they can do something, the next moment they can't—or won't. Assuming this is only a case of stubbornness, caregivers insist that loved ones try harder. Sometimes the person does better, reinforcing the caregivers' belief that trying harder works—however, trying harder is not always an option.

Alzheimer's victims may be overwhelmed by demands that become threatening to them. First, they may not be aware of or understand what is expected of them. They may not know what to do or how to do it today, even though they knew yesterday. The emotional message communicated by caregivers may upset and confuse them, and distract their attention from tasks at hand.

Resulting confusion   Finally, individuals may not even be aware of their impairments. Their response to demands may be reduced to anger, tears, or even greater stubbornness. They may be confused because they don't understand the task or why they must do it. They may be able to sense the caregiver's frustration, yet not understand its source.

Even though you may be in doubt, it generally is best to assume loved ones are trying as hard as they can. There might be other ways to get them to complete a task or improve their behavior. There is a saying employers often share with employees who may be working furiously but failing to accomplish enough: "Work smarter, not harder." This can be applied to Alzheimer's care. Pressing the Alzheimer's victim to work harder may create a catastrophic reaction. As a caregiver, you can work smarter by trying other approaches, backing off for awhile, or changing your mind about how important it is for this particular thing to be done right now.

Emotions and Alzheimer's Behavior

Caregivers often wonder how loved ones perceive emotions. The fact that their intellectual abilities are diminishing does not necessarily mean they cannot experience a wide range of emotions, or be aware of the emotional content of what you express to them. In many cases, they may be "more" sensitive to what is communicated emotionally. Their own emotional expressions may reflect their reactions to what is happening at a particular moment, or represent the more persistent feelings they experience from time to time, such as, fear, anger, anxiety, embarrassment, or different faces of confusion.

Emotions are messages   Displays of negative emotions like these may be uncomfortable for you as the caregiver. They may signal that something you are doing is distressing, or that they fail to comprehend what is expected of them. Negative emotions may suggest something unpleasant or stressful in your environment. For instance, it is too dark, too noisy, too cold, or too hot. Perhaps the normal daily routine has been changed. Furniture may have been moved, or something else may have changed in what had been a familiar place. This is disconcerting and creates a greater sense of insecurity for the person with Alzheimer's. Persons with brain impairment have greater difficulty adjusting to changes.

As caregivers become more familiar with how their own behaviors and certain aspects of the physical environment affect loved ones emotionally, they can change what and how things are being done. Perhaps they need to slow down and be more encouraging. The music that was enjoyable for a little while becomes irritating if it continues. Unpleasant activities like bathing may be difficult to get started. Once the resistance has faded, this type of activity can be positive. On the other hand, behavioral or emotional problems in loved ones can suggest something "internal" is bothering them, which has nothing to do with you or the external environment.

Negative emotions might also indicate that loved ones are more aware of changes in themselves. At times, denial or being unaware of the changes protects them from what must be an awesome realization. When they recognize that they cannot remember well, are unable to do things right, or don't know what to do, their behavior and emotional reactions may be more negative. Their caregivers may be perplexed or frightened by these situations. They may feel helpless in knowing their loved ones are experiencing emotions that are the result of disturbing, but inaccessible perceptions.

Emotions and behaviors as clues

These emotions may reflect their loved ones' grief over the loss of their abilities and themselves. They may experience regret about their dependence upon you and the burden they have become. They may be fearful of being left alone to face a process they are quite unable to stop. Worst of all, those persons for whom caregivers have so much concern might be unable to verbalize their fears and confusion. The thoughts are locked in; caregivers are locked out. Therefore, the best clues in helping caregivers understand their loved ones are the emotions and behaviors they observe in them.

Not all emotional reactions are negative. Positive emotions are also experienced by your loved one. Many of the same activities and experiences that used to stimulate positive emotions may still produce pleasant reactions. Your wife or husband's emotional reaction to something still depends upon their perception and understanding of it. If we don't catch the humor in a joke someone tells us, we are not likely to laugh even though it is expected of us. If other people are laughing outrageously, we might chuckle, but we still don't understand what is so funny. On the other hand, if some scene in a movie touches us in a sad way we might become tearful and cry. Other people may not have perceived that scene the way we did. Their experiences may have been different, or they simply did not understand things the way we did.

Individual emotional factors

The emotional reactions of Alzheimer's victims are still influenced by their individual characteristics. Family members must remember that affected loved ones are no longer as perceptive and do not perceive many situations as clearly as they may have in the past. They are unable to understand what is happening as well. Instead of becoming more involved in activities or situations that were previously enjoyable, they might withdraw more as familiar situations become confusing.

Situational influences   If—on the basis of their understanding of behavior—family members can accommodate relatives in activities, their brain-impaired relatives have a better chance of following what is happening. Simple and clearer explanations of what is going on, and how it applies to them, enhance their chances of enjoying situations. Expectations are more specific and attainable. Alzheimer's victims may not be able to perceive the "whole" situation, but they can at least feel more appropriately involved.

Social situations created by family get-togethers may produce overwhelming mental and emotional stimulation. Making such situations more comprehensible for your loved one also reduces his own emotional reactions to the behavior of others around him. For instance, when a caregiving daughter invites other family members to dinner, her father will probably relate better to this situation if she can intercede on his behalf. For example, if two people are speaking to him at once, he will likely become more anxious and confused. Rather than be able to say, "I can't answer everybody at once," he may walk away or become more irritated than the situation would have normally suggested. He might tell everyone to leave. He could perceive he is doing something wrong, or "messing up." The Alzheimer's victim might seem more suspicious to family members unaccustomed to the changes he has undergone in their absence.

Emotions and morale   Positive emotional expressions have very positive effects on caregivers. Laughter, smiles, responses of humor, and expressions of affection are always welcomed. For that matter, the absence of negative emotion is readily accepted. Positive emotions and the absence of negative emotions give us the impression that our loved one is feeling fine and not suffering so much. If those we care for are not distressed and seem satisfied with what is going on for the moment, our burdens are lightened a bit.

Caregivers cannot easily separate themselves from the emotional responses of their relatives. A relationship exists and many interactions are bound to it. We are sensitive to the emotional expressions of loved ones because they help us understand the relationship. Alzheimer's disease does more than affect one spouse or parent. It impacts all relationships. It affects everyone in the family. Just as patterns of behavior existed prior to Alzheimer's disease, patterns of emotional reactions also existed. Recognition of these patterns were an important means of knowing your loved one. For a time, these reactions can still be predicted because they are still a part of your loved one's personality.

The aspects of relationships that involve the intellect and thinking tend to diminish early in the disease process. Social aspects of relationships, particularly intimacy, are gradually lost. Caregivers often remain intensely involved in efforts to sustain some semblance of the relationships they have had with the victims. Their efforts are constantly threatened by the victim's behavioral changes, the presence of psychiatric symptoms such as delusions, angry or hostile behavior directed at them, and the discouraging advice of others. The absence of encouragement and appreciation from their relative is all too obvious.

Emotional and Behavioral Communication

All of us like to know that what we do is appreciated. We all benefit from encouragement, especially when the challenge may be greater than our physical and emotional resources. Caregivers must expect less encouragement and appreciation from loved ones affected by Alzheimer's since their world is being diminished by loss of memory, the capacity to think, and the ability to relate to others as appropriately as they had before the disease became more pronounced. These changes in brain function ultimately contribute to severe errors of social judgment. These errors are not the result of "ill intentions," although they may appear so at times.

Feedback as aid to communication When we interact with people it's helpful to know how effectively we are communicating with them. Feedback tells us how the other person is receiving what we are saying or doing: does he understand what you mean, does she like what you are doing. Emotional expressions, the way the person acts, or what the person says are all sources of feedback. We can modify what we say or do on the basis of this information. He or she will be less likely to give you much verbal information unless you ask questions. You may be able to get some type of yes or no response to simple questions, if what you are asking is understood by your family member. These responses may add only to your confusion, rather than your understanding of what did or did not happen. Since verbal behavior becomes less reliable and understandable in Alzheimer's patients, caregivers must rely on other aspects of communication for feedback.

Emotional reactions and behavior of those for whom we care become more important sources of feedback for caregivers. Negative emotional reactions may tell you that you are asking too much, or expecting it too quickly. Anxious or agitated behavior suggests your loved ones may become more upset unless you modify your expectations and become more supportive and encouraging. When your husband passively resists a request to get up and go to the kitchen, he may not understand your request or be sure how to get to the kitchen. He might feel ashamed about this and depend on you to guide him to the kitchen. Emotional and behavioral messages provide caregivers with important clues for managing behavior. Caregivers who fail to recognize and interpret these clues appropriately may be inviting the occurrence of a catastrophic reaction, a phenomena that is common in brain damaged individuals and predicted by recognition of specific emotional and behavioral signs. We will consider this phenomena shortly.

There is a scene in the video production of "Caregiving with Grace" (Cohen and Whitford 1987) that illustrates our points about behavior, emotional reactions to experiences, the effects of the disease on relationships, and the need caregivers have for some small sign of appreciation. "Caregiving with Grace" reflects the changes in Grace's behavior and abilities about ten years after Alzheimer's had been diagnosed. Her husband, Glen, demonstrates how he interacts and works with his wife when providing the assistance necessary for activities of daily living to be completed. Rather than simply doing these activities for Grace, Glen tries to involve her in some part of the task.

Glen is painting his wife's fingernails. It is about 3:00 in the afternoon, and though Glen is a model caregiver with an exemplary understanding of the disease's effects on Grace's behavior, he has related the frustrations he experiences daily. He recognizes the fact that Grace cannot be expected to express her gratitude for what he does. In fact her emotional expressions seem anxious and tense during this experience of having her fingernails painted. Glen is not just painting her fingernails; he is repeatedly encouraging Grace to participate in this activity in small but significant ways. "Hold still." "Give me this hand." He also gives Grace feedback about how she is doing and how nice she looks with her fingernails painted. Finally his task is done, and he both asks and shows Grace how to wave her hands in the air so they will dry quicker.

Grace looks pleased and relieved. Perhaps she is pleased with how her fingernails look, and that she had some involvement in the completion of this activity. They completed something as a couple. She is certainly relieved by the decrease of demands on her. Then Glen invites her to thank him for what he has done. She appears a little perplexed. Maybe she thought everything was finished, yet now she must say "Thank You" when she had not uttered a word all day. Glen persists with encouragement. The emotional expressions on her face indicate she is trying. She makes sounds that are a closer approximation of frustration than "Thank You." Suddenly the viewer witnesses a victory. The words come forth. Her facial expressions suggest she has accomplished something. Despite the fact it was solicited, she gave something to her husband. Something that suggests more about a relationship than it does the completion of a task.

Behavior and Stress

Caregivers less familiar with how to perform an activity with a relative whose impaired memory creates deficits in behavior might have been more reluctant than Glen to continue. Without understanding why, they could have anticipated the situation to worsen. Instead of completing the desired task, they could have been confronted by more difficult behavioral problems in their loved ones. Both would then be involved in a progressively more sensitive and stressful situation. Some activities of daily living, for example, dressing, bathing, eating, and toileting, need to be completed. One time may be better than another, but Alzheimer's victims eventually do not remember why one does these things. Caregivers experience a good deal of stress from the anticipated behavioral and emotional reactions loved ones might exhibit when they are trying to finish simple activities of daily living.

Stress as predictor of problems

Glen was very attentive to Grace's behavior and emotional expressions. They were good measures of how stressful having her fingernails painted was for her. Glen gauged how firm and encouraging he needed to be on the basis of behavioral and emotional clues. He did not require too much of Grace, though at times she became more anxious. His own emotional reaction was calm, which matched the content of his verbal encouragement. His approach prevented her from overreacting to minor stressors.

The stress experienced by persons with Alzheimer's and the way they behave and function is closely related. Their anxiety will serve as a fairly reliable indicator of how much activity and stimulation they can tolerate. They are quite responsive to reductions of stress in their environments; the more impaired they are, the more strongly their environments influence the outcomes of their interactions (Lawton 1989). In this sense, environment is more than the physical setting in which these persons live. Environment involves their interactions with people and things, and even their responses to their own thoughts.

Multiple and simultaneous messages or distractions are two examples of stressors that Alzheimer's victims experience. Nonverbal messages that pressure them to hurry are stressful, as are commands that carry the same message. Any demands that are placed on areas of impaired cognitive functioning will increase their experience of stress. Other sources of stress include pressure to perform tasks that are complex because they have multiple steps, illness, not being understood or being able to understand, fatigue, frustration, fear, anxiety, or perceiving nonverbal negative messages. Receiving negative verbal messages can be stressful and demoralizing to these individuals. Their own awareness of their mistakes and impairments is probably a fairly persistent source of stress.

Stress reduction as a tool

Caregivers need to pay careful attention to other sources of stress that individuals experience and remove or diminish the strength of such stressors. Brain damage itself does not sufficiently explain many of the behavior difficulties you and your loved one experience. Situations that are overly stressful can have much to do with these problems. If you minimize stressors, you reduce the possibility of more severe behavioral and emotional outbursts.

Catastrophic Reactions

Stress, fear, fatigue, and anxiety are common experiences for people with Alzheimer's disease. Everyone of us has a "breaking point." We are already dealing with more stress than we thought we could handle. It only takes another small demand on us and we "blow." From one day to the next that breaking point may change, depending on how much stress we are under at the time. Brain-damaged individuals cannot tolerate the amount of stress they used to handle. "Small things" can become "big things." When brain-damaged individuals overreact to minor stressors, they exhibit "catastrophic" reactions. "Little things" are overwhelming.

What is meant by catastrophic reactions has already been shown in the examples in this chapter. They include behaviors and emotional reactions that are as common as they are disturbing. Catastrophic reactions are manifested as angry outbursts, refusals to do something, agitation, pacing, more intense anxiety, tearfulness, whining, mumbling, or even crying. In more extreme cases, catastrophic reactions may include hitting or striking out.

Too often the assertion that persons with Alzheimer's disease are aggressive results from a poor understanding of catastrophic reactions. Persons with Alzheimer's disease are already overwhelmed and their choices of protective responses are reduced to basic "fight" or "flight." If they are cornered during catastrophic reactions, these individuals often try to withdraw. Their other response to these feelings is likely to be defensive, but it is labeled aggressive by those who misinterpret it, thus, making it worse.

The behavioral and emotional changes associated with catastrophic reactions usually build in intensity, but they can appear suddenly and be quite intense. Catastrophic reactions may occur infrequently and seem to be unpredictable and sporadic. They may also occur almost continuously, and environmental or interpersonal factors that encourage them can be identified. Some sources may be very simple, such as asking a person to do more than they are capable of doing or asking too many questions. A new situation, person, or environment can precipitate catastrophic reactions. Some source of confusion or insecurity is often involved. It may take a combination of factors to precipitate these reactions one day, and many fewer factors the next. The reactions are largely beyond the control of the person exhibiting them.

Easier to pre-
vent than stop
Alzheimer's caregivers need to attend to potential sources of anxiety, fear, fatigue, and stress
since it is much easier to prevent catastrophic reactions than stop them in progress (Mace 1990).
While catastrophic reactions are common with this disease, their
sources are often a function of the individual preferences of the person experiencing them. An activity or situation may be comfortable
for one individual but become quite threatening to another. For example, some persons can tolerate being alone; others cling to
caregivers whenever there is an indication they might be left alone.

Excess Disability

Caregivers may notice that loved ones are not functioning as well as
they could realistically expect. Some fluctuations in behavior can be
anticipated because of the progressive but sometimes unpredictable
progression of this disease. However, some impairment or disability
may not be attributable to the disease. This has been called "excess
disability" and has many potential sources during the course of this
disease.

In Alzheimer's disease, excess disability can commonly be attributed to the presence of other illnesses, medications, psychiatric
symptoms related to the disease, sensory impairments such as poor
vision and hearing, stress, fatigue, and anxiety (Mace 1990). Care
environments that encourage unnecessary dependency foster excess
disability. Social or physical environments that have too little stimulation have the same result. Caregivers must take the presence of excess disability very seriously, and whenever possible see that it is
eliminated or reduced. This may require professional assistance. The
result is certainly worthwhile. Loved ones might be able to function
better and more appropriately. This in turn reduces the additional
stress you as a caregiver, experience, and those for who you care
might feel better about themselves.

Summary

Behavioral changes associated with the experience of Alzheimer's disease have many sources. Brain damage is only one source of change

in behavior and the behavior management problems caregivers must face. Understanding the changes that occur through the stages of the disease process might help family caregivers appreciate some of the changes they may encounter. Like so many aspects of Alzheimer's disease, stages are a rough guide. They map how behavior "might change," providing a general sense of what you can expect, but you must be ready to respond to changes when the map is wrong. Behavior is the result of a dynamic pattern of responses to stimuli that produce action, feelings, and thoughts. Individual personality, the severity of brain impairment, the physical and interpersonal environment, and many other factors influence how people perceive and respond to stimulation outside themselves.

Beliefs about behavior   Emotional and behavioral reactions can be traced to the thoughts and feelings relatives experience. Many of the ideas we have considered have application to the behavior of caregivers themselves. Beliefs caregivers have about behavior influence their own understanding and reactions to it. It will be necessary to change beliefs that fail to account for the impact of brain damage on behavior. It is important to better understand the relationship between behavior and brain damage.

Brain damage influences the ways persons with Alzheimer's disease understand and perceive things. It affects how these individuals act and react. Their behavior and emotional reactions to experiences will gradually suggest more of the impact of the disease, and both will provide clues that suggest how the caregiver can manage the situation. They provide the caregiver with information about what to do and not to do. Recognizing this helps "head off" a catastrophic reaction, and reduce the stress of the situation—yours and his.

Emotions—negative and positive—influence behavior and the way afflicted people can think and remember. Their behavior and personality will fit together in less predictable ways. These changes will have dramatic effects on what they can do and require you, as their caregivers, to do more for them.

Environments play a key role in the way victims of Alzheimer's function. Physical and social environments must be adapted so that they are less confusing and overwhelming, more secure and familiar. The environment must be comfortable and supportive of caregiving and daily living. While these environments need to provide stimulation, they cannot provide so much they significantly exceed the coping abilities of loved ones. The behavior and emotional reactions of loved ones progressively become determined more by their environments and the persons in those environments.

Excess disabilities created by conditions like depression and other health problems must be addressed so that the functioning of individuals experiencing the mental, emotional, and eventually physical manifestations of this disease is not further compromised.

Within these changes, there are many losses. But these losses cannot be experienced only as losses of behavior. They represent the losses of relationships, the losses of persons you love. Caregivers are compelled to care for someone they love with very little encouragement. The more they care for the person, the more they realize that the person is leaving. This departure seems never to be finished and one feels suspended in a moment of grief that constantly repeats itself.

Glimpses of the person Understanding behavioral changes helps caregivers appreciate those small glimmers of the old personality that appear through the long days of caring. Someone "is" still there, and must be trying just as you are trying. A small step is not much, but it might remind you of a moment when you were walking together, and the relationship you once had is again present. Little things can make a big difference.

As a relative who has become the caregiver for someone with Alzheimer's disease, you will be tempted to feel solely responsible for all of the problems that arise during the course of the disease. We must not forget that loved ones, too, are often struggling to do something about what is happening to them. The changes that you may witness that are unacceptable and cause greater concern may represent another glimmer of personality. They may represent the efforts of loved ones to adapt to what is so difficult to understand and accept. When that is the case, it is something you share. You are both trying to understand and accept the changes.

ACCEPTANCE

You have Alzheimer's disease
and you're losing the power
to remember—to reason—to understand,
to do the simple tasks
we take for granted:
to put on a shoe—
to button a shirt—
to read a book—
to remember a face or name.

It's a hard thing to understand—
to accept . . . . .
Perhaps it's been the hardest for me,
for I've lived with you—
but I know—you can't help it—
can't act otherwise . . . .

I must take you as you are
and expect—not more—but less
as the disease continues to progress.

Maude S. Newton

8

STAGES OF FAMILY ADJUSTMENT

We must find a way to accept the disease. Adjusting to the reality of Alzheimer's disease in a loved one is a complex and difficult process. Yet we must find a way to reconcile ourselves to the disease as best we can, for accepting the disease makes it easier to handle the emotional and physical strains that Alzheimer's brings. If we continue to deny the disease and its implications, we risk denying both the victim and ourselves the support and care that are needed.

Adjusting to Alzheimer's is like adjusting to a death. Because Alzheimer's is a fatal disease and one that often involves a lingering death, the stages of grief that family members go through are very similar to the stages of adjustment to death described by Dr. Elizabeth Kübler-Ross in her 1969 book, *On Death and Dying.* It is useful to understand these stages, both as they correspond to one's own psychological adjustment to the disease and for the light they may shed on the reactions of other family members.

Each individual finds her own way to become reconciled to the disease. Not everyone will go through these stages in the same way, of course, and some family members will find it easier to accept the disease than others. Each individual will probably find that she can reconcile herself to what is happening at some times better than others. Often we may misinterpret the reactions of those around us or wish they would adjust differently. If family members accept the idea that each person must face up to the disease in his own way, however, the family can serve as a strong support system throughout the adjustment process.

We must be understanding of the adjustment process of others.
In one family, for example, a mother and her son may react very differently to the illness of the father. The mother may feel a helpless anger and compensate by becoming overly involved with the illness, shutting out her son. The son may feel abandoned by his father and snubbed by his mother and may lash out in frustration when she refuses to let him help. Rather than make things more difficult for each other, both mother and son must work to understand the other's adjustment process and to accept it, as long as serious questions of sufficient care or the caregiver's health are not involved.

In considering the family's stages of acceptance, it is important to remember the following facts.

- Each family member must have the chance to work through the stages of grief to final acceptance of the disease. This does not mean that encouragement and support are not needed, nor that professional help is not indicated.

- What family members are willing to do about the loved one's needs and their own is influenced by where they are in the adjustment process. Caregiving is not simply a mechanical experience; it also involves one's thoughts and feelings.

- The adjustment process does not always occur in clearly defined stages. Long-standing conflicts and repressed feelings may need resolving before acceptance can be reached. In such cases, professional counseling may be advisable.

Kübler-Ross' stages of acceptance
The following are Dr. Kübler-Ross' stages of adjustment to death.

1. **Denial and isolation.** The person experiences shocked disbelief when faced with imminent death. She thinks: "No, this can't happen to me . . . it can't be true!"

2. **Anger and resentment.** The person's thoughts revolve around "Why me?" and "What have I done to deserve this?" She feels anger and bitterness toward others, the world, and even herself.

3. **Bargaining.** In her mind, the person tries to buy back her life with some promise or action. "I'll do anything if you'll give me another day, a year, five years," she may think. God may be called on in the bargaining to heal the person and restore life.

4. **Depression.** The person despairingly gives in to death because it cannot be stopped. "What's the use?" she thinks. "Why go on fighting?"

5. **Acceptance.** The person withdraws into peace and a final rest.

While these reactions are generally experienced by the dying person, family members may experience them as well.

The stages defined by Kübler-Ross do not entail all that is involved in one's acceptance of death. Some persons may never accept death. They may die still angry that life has cheated them. A spouse may be depressed for months after the death and remain angry even longer.

Perception of loss is an individual experience. It is not appropriate to compare one family's loss with the losses of others. However, some families may be affected by the following factors that make their loss especially difficult to accept.

1. **The age of the person when Alzheimer's is diagnosed.** Younger victims forced to leave their jobs must contend with loss of income and insurance benefits. The healthy spouse may still be working, which makes arranging for caregiving more difficult.

2. **The general health of the victim.** When the Alzheimer's victim is in otherwise good health, the feeling of being cheated by life may be more intense. A person may have been prepared for cancer or heart disease but not a mysterious illness like Alzheimer's.

3. **The length of the illness.** The emotional strains of extended caregiving, along with its physical and financial costs, may intensify the family's feeling of abandonment and loss.

4. **The family's expectations.** Alzheimer's disease may be nothing like the family imagined, or the family may feel disappointed in the response of health professionals to their loved one's condition.

5. **The family's emotional closeness.** The afflicted person's loss of social and intellectual capabilities creates tremendous barriers to communication, and some families may not be able to counteract their sense of separation and isolation from the person.

6. **Preexisting family roles.** The spouse affected by Alzheimer's may have been responsible for managing most, if not all, of the family's affairs. The manifestations of the illness create a greater threat to the spouse-caregiver when she must assume the new duties of family management plus caregiving.

Adjustment to the disease usually includes five stages.

The following stages of family adjustment are based upon the stages identified by Kübler-Ross but have been modified by Paul Teusink and Susan Mahler (see Bibliography) to reflect the normal series of responses that families go through when confronted by Alzheimer's disease.

1. **Denial.** Reflects the initial response that nothing is wrong.

2. **Overinvolvement.** Similar to bargaining; represents an attempt to compensate for the illness and associated impairments.

3. **Anger.** Follows when the family realizes that compensation has failed.

4. **Guilt.** Develops out of the anger and "what ifs" precipitated by looking back.

5. **Acceptance.** Resolution or acceptance of the problems.

Each of these stages will be treated in depth.

1. Denial

Denial is a natural reaction.

Denial is the most common and frequently used defense, and it comes into play from the beginning. Beliefs about senility and old age lead the family to excuse the victim's forgetfulness and thus help to sustain denial. Family members really may not feel certain that anything serious is wrong.

Denial can create dangerous situations.

Denying the problem allows family members to postpone action. When the person lives alone, children may resist evaluating what is happening. Neighbors or friends may call to report some concerns; children may visit the parent to check these reports. However, their own denial prevents them from doing more than visiting more frequently or encouraging the parent to get out and do more.

The denial also prevents the family from adequately recognizing or facing the extent of the impairment and its consequences. The family's failure to understand such consequences places the loved one in a higher risk situation, particularly if she is living alone.

Denial can create family conflict.

Some family members may recognize that action needs to be taken but encounter denial from other family members. If a family leader is denying the problem, it can be more difficult for the others to get professional help for the affected relative.

Denying symptoms is a normal defense against threats to one's well-being. It is normal and necessary to gradually adjust to the implications of the disease. The slow progression of the illness provides time for the family to make this adjustment and to accept what is happening.

Denial creates barriers to care and family involvement.

Excessive denial can be quite destructive, however. It blocks help and any movement toward acceptance. Plans for care cannot be made until a realistic assessment of the patient's and the family's needs is made.

Moving past denial

The following steps will help families to move past denial:

- Seeking and receiving information about Alzheimer's disease and the family experience
- Getting a professional evaluation of the victim's degree of impairment
- Understanding the consequences of the impairment and, with professional assistance, becoming sensitive to the patient's reactions to the illness
- Seeking counseling with a professional if denial is excessive
- Addressing issues emerging from the denial with personal, family, and professional support.

A thorough evaluation of the patient's condition involves numerous health professionals.

During the actual evaluation process, it is quite appropriate for families to seek a second opinion. However, seeking many opinions can indicate desperate denial. In most situations, the Alzheimer's diagnosis already involves several opinions. For example, the following evaluative process is used at DePaul Center, a psychiatric hospital in Waco, Texas. Such a process addresses the need for a comprehensive evaluation to effectively plan activities involving the patient, family, and community resources.

Medical evaluation. Includes basic tests (e.g., blood chemistry, chest Xray, electrocardiogram, etc.) and specified elective tests (e.g., EEG or brain scan). Additionally, a neurologist or other specialists may be consulted.

Psychiatric evaluation. Assesses the presence of other psychiatric illnesses consistent with symptoms, such as severe depression; considers medications' effects and utilization as well as other medical findings.

Social history. Includes psychosocial history and assessment of the family system, resources available, and resources needed.

Psychological/Neuropsychological testing. Assists in differentiating strengths and weaknesses related to dementia and a person's emotional reactions to it; identifies actual deficits related to impaired brain function or other psychiatric disorders.

Therapy evaluation. A physical therapist and occupational therapist evaluate functioning and determine rehabilitation needs and potential.

Even when family members seem to accept the diagnosis of Alzheimer's disease, denial may leave them vulnerable to shopping for cures or believing that medication prescribed to manage symptoms will cure the disease.

False hopes   Sometimes, denial reemerges when there seem to be fluctuations in the person's condition. Good days seem to promise the person is improving. Bad days intensify the family's worries that the person is deteriorating rapidly. Families can profit most by getting off the emotional roller coaster of alternating hope and despair, while making the most of the good days.

2. Overinvolvement

Stage two of the family reaction is overinvolvement. The primary caregiver may try to meet every need of the affected person, become severely isolated, and refuse assistance or support from any source. Often, the individual demonstrating overinvolvement is a spouse, although families as a whole can be overinvolved as well.

**Overinvolve-
ment seeks to
counter the
impact of
the illness.**   Once family members overcome the denial stage and admit to themselves that the illness exists, they naturally want to take action. For the family of an Alzheimer's patient, active involvement with the victim represents a way to attempt to counteract the effects of the illness and compensate for their relative's losses. The impact of the

illness can be made less noticeable when the family is covering for the relative in all areas.

Overinvolve-ment can spur families into action.

A family's overinvolvement can become a tool for providing the best possible care to the afflicted relative. As this stage begins, the family can plan their involvement in the overall care. Particular attention should be paid to support for the Alzheimer's victim and her spouse, who very likely will become overinvolved. Overinvolvement is a form of bargaining. When compensations fail, other strong emotions emerge.

Overinvolve-ment can create barriers to asking for help.

Overinvolvement becomes dangerous, however, when it reaches extreme proportions. Many persons who become overinvolved fail to seek help when they should. Loyalty, duty, family, and cultural values, combined with a strong sense of obligation, reinforce the view that the caregiver must handle the illness alone. Nonetheless, such individuals reach a point when they are more open to help, even though they may not ask for it directly.

Extreme overinvolvement can lead to greater isolation and to the caregiver's sacrificing herself to the illness. Examples of caregivers who have experienced major health problems, such as high blood pressure and stress-related illnesses, are common.

Help for the overinvolved caregiver

The following is an outline to follow in helping the overinvolved caregiver.

- Explore and discuss available options. A caregiver may accept the need for help in the home before she can consider institutionalization.
- Involve other family members and friends in different aspects of the care situation.
- Help the caregiver to relinquish the burden of guilt by pointing out that the patient's needs have surpassed the resources of any one person.

- If true, emphasize that the type of care needed cannot successfully be provided in the home setting.

- Help the caregiver to realize that her overinvolvement is hurting both the patient and herself, and is likely creating problems for the rest of the family.

- Suggest that lessening the spouse's care load may improve the quality of time she spends with the loved one.

3. Anger

The third stage of the acceptance process is anger, which can stem from the added physical and emotional burden caused by continued deterioration in the person and the caregiving situation. The caregiver's dedication and sacrifices may not seem to have made any difference. Also, the resources needed may not be available or may cost more than the family can afford.

Angry reactions cause guilt. Caregivers who have been tolerant of their relative's embarrassing behavior may begin to get angry as the behavior moves beyond their control. In turn, the loss of control may precipitate guilt feelings. Unfortunately, some family members lose even more control under intense stress and verbally and/or physically abuse the loved one.

Anger can stem from feelings of abandonment. The family can feel angry about being abandoned by the clearly dysfunctional relative, which can be further complicated by long-standing interpersonal problems. Whether justified or not, a caregiver may be hostile toward family and friends. Feelings of being left alone and having to make all the decisions by oneself can intensify anger. However, angry outbursts should be avoided, as they can alienate family members from one another. The anger stage of acceptance may leave the primary caregiver and others in the family quite sensitive to critical remarks about the care decisions they have made.

Misdirected anger is common. While a person is in the anger stage, her reactions can touch others who have been less directly involved with in-home caregiving. Staff members in long-term care facilities need to recognize that anger is a part of the road to acceptance. However, family members should recognize and address its real source. Otherwise, it can be misdirected toward persons who are crucial to the loved one's care or others who play vital roles in supporting the family.

4. Guilt

Guilt is a normal reaction to Alzheimer's. However, those involved must take care that the powerful combination of unresolved anger and guilt they feel does not become overwhelming and develop into serious depression. (See Chapter 3.) Caregivers may need professional help to resolve unrelenting feelings of anger and guilt.

Guilt can arise from old conflicts. Much guilt can arise from family conflicts left unresolved over the years. Family members may dwell on past regrets, wishing they could only do things over. Relatives may find themselves dwelling on such questions as "What if an evaluation had been done a year sooner?" or "What if we had seen another doctor?" They may think "We should have done more for her and spent more time with her while she was healthy." But the family must eventually put aside such thoughts, forgive themselves, and go on living.

Guilt about the wish for death It is not uncommon for family members to wish that their loved one would die and then feel guilty about that wish. As hard as it is to lose someone, most persons can view death in the last stage of Alzheimer's disease as a real blessing for their loved one and for those who cared so much for so long.

Regrets can become overwhelming.

Guilt also can be triggered by the caregiver's angry acts or imagined omissions. Perhaps she did not do enough, or perhaps she lashed out at her relative in frustration. But the caregiver must not let regrets and guilt overwhelm her; it is only human to occasionally lose control under such stressful circumstances.

Other sources of guilt

Family members often find themselves giving their relative with Alzheimer's information that is not completely true. They may tell their relative they are taking her to the store, when the destination is really the doctor's office. They may not be truthful about the purpose of a medication for delusions or agitation. These "white lies" are sometimes a source of guilt because family members believe they are being dishonest with their loved one, tricking her or lying to her. It is best to remember the motivations behind these actions.

Half-truths and caring

Half-truths may be necessary for appropriate care or to help families manage their affected relatives. Persons with Alzheimer's disease fail to understand the logic behind many actions as their illness progresses. Attempts to reason with them will only make matters worse in many cases. If they become extremely agitated and resistant, taking medication or trips to the doctor can become major caregiving stressors. Family members need not feel guilty about many of the half-truths they use to care for their loved ones.

Tough decisions can create guilt.

Decisions made against the wishes of the patient can leave the caregiver struggling with feelings of guilt. If a spouse or child forced the visit to the doctor, she may feel guilt after the evaluation confirming the diagnosis of Alzheimer's. Likewise, placing her loved one in a nursing home or another institution can raise doubts and feelings of guilt. Hopefully, this conflict can be handled by realizing that the loved one's needs cannot be provided for at home. Most likely, the caregiver already has done all she could and given much more of herself than she would have thought possible.

5. Acceptance

The fight is over. Acceptance, the final stage of a family's response to Alzheimer's disease, is possible when the process of the disease and its effect on others is fully understood. It is easier once the family members have found within themselves the resources to cope with Alzheimer's. Resources in the community become a part of their strength and are accepted in turn once they fully comprehend the impact of the illness.

The anger and guilt associated with each person's adjustment is now behind her, and she can see each stage's place in moving toward a more peaceful acceptance of fate. She can recognize, without reservation, that her loved one is no longer the person she once knew.

New situations can precipitate a return or regression to earlier stages of adjustment. The need to let go of unfinished plans or dreams, or the comments of friends and family may trigger a temporary setback. The caregiver should understand that such experiences are simply brief detours, rather than roadblocks in the adjustment process.

9

FAMILY RESPONSES TO CARE

The experience of grief is a significant part of the family adjustment to Alzheimer's disease. Victims of the disease know something bad is happening. Our understanding of how these persons grieve is imperfect. Some behavioral and emotional problems may be manifestations of their grief. The family caregiver and other relatives experience stress and strain that directly relate to the grief experience. They also experience stress resulting from failure of the family to support the tasks of caregiving—the interactions that provide for the needs of the chronically affected relative on an unrelenting, daily basis. Alzheimer's disease creates a crisis in a family.

The losses that reflect the progressive deterioration of a individual suggest the loss of the family as it was known. Gradually it becomes apparent that the roles played by the relative with Alzheimer's disease can no longer be managed by that individual. Other family members must assume some of these responsibilities. The wife, for example, may find herself responsible for decisions that her husband would ordinarily have made. Even though she may now make these decisions, his influence may still be considerable. In more extreme cases, the Alzheimer's spouse—even while suffering the more advanced manifestations of the disease—may actually be involved in decision making.

Need for family support The influence of other family members and friends will be critical in helping caregivers to takeover and control activities such as driving and making financial decisions. Often, the family caregiver will not prevent the loved one with Alzheimer's from driving, carelessly paying bills, or making extravagant purchases. In other families, the children would prevent any opportunity for the afflicted person to drive or handle money. Their response might be so forceful that it causes more emotional difficulties in the family. One child might be willing to intervene in certain family matters, but stay away from other situations. Another child may choose to stay away from family interactions altogether.

Roles change Part of the family adjustment to the crisis of Alzheimer's disease involves changes in normal family roles. Pre-existing patterns of interacting and communicating will have considerable influence on how families address these changes. These changes can be quite difficult or even impossible to make. In others, they seem to be made with relative ease. Families are unique. In some families, changes are too unsettling, even when they would support the stability of the family and the needs of the affected relative and his caregiver.

More directly than other family members, the primary family caregiver will experience the successes and failures of family responses to the needs created by Alzheimer's disease. Expectations of family members need to be tempered with an understanding of how they have responded to previous crises in the family. Consider the various roles different family members have assumed, the quality of their support, and their willingness to be involved. In short, family members need to re-evaluate how they interact with one another. When all family members are together, the atmosphere and quality of the interaction may be quite different.

There are several ways one can consider family interactions during times of crises. We will examine some characteristics of different family interactions (Blazer 1984). The quality of interactions in these descriptions of family characteristics varies considerably. Several characteristics apply to families and influence their effectiveness in dealing with the stress of caregiving as a healthy family unit.

Compatible vs. Conflictual Families

Family interactions are compatible when members usually agree with one another. Small differences can exist, but are usually reconciled without much apparent disagreement. Interactions that reveal conflict and more obvious differences are more likely to impede family attempts to develop clear, unified responses to problems. Some conflict may be desirable. An extremely compatible family may be afraid of conflict. To avoid conflict, major issues may be ignored. Compatible family interactions are likely to promote a more relaxed atmosphere that further fosters working together; highly conflictual family interactions create an atmosphere of tension, anxiety, anger, and hurt. The tasks of caregiving are frustrated by interpersonal conflicts.

Crises like Alzheimer's disease have the capacity to stimulate conflict. All family members are affected. The future of the family and its members may become uncertain. Such a situation affects relationships and changes them. These changes in relationships among parents and children have been referred to as "rejoining" (Blazer 1984). Rejoining parents and children can be difficult because of some of the conflicts that arise. There are three types of conflict that can occur when a crisis affects changes in the parent/child relationship during rejoining: continuing, new, and reactivated.

Continuing conflicts

Continuing conflicts have always been present between parents and their children. When Alzheimer's disease develops, new problems face the family. Adult daughters may feel compelled to become more involved than their own immediate family responsibilities would seem to allow. However, their reason for declining the responsibility of hands-on care for a parent may be supported by old, unresolved conflicts, not competing family duties. Perhaps the parent with Alzheimer's disease was the parent who drank too much and had been abusive. Continuing conflicts that involve a history of abuse can predict risks in Alzheimer's caregiving when the abused child is faced with caring for the abusive parent. The expectation of reasonable give-and-take between parents and children might have been violated and represent the source of continuing conflict.

Continuing conflicts may interfere with new problems being addressed in Alzheimer's care. The unfinished business they reflect needs to be resolved if at all possible. If it involves the parent now afflicted with Alzheimer's, it needs to be completed before the intellectual impairment surpasses the person's capacity to participate in the problem-solving process. Alzheimer's disease can affect all family members in continuing conflicts.

New conflicts   *New* conflicts may develop in families confronted by Alzheimer's disease and reflect issues that never required attention before. These crises are normal for well-adjusted families (Blazer 1984), and relate to issues concerning nursing home placement, death and dying, living arrangements, the type of professional help that might be needed, and the distribution of family resources and responsibilities. These issues may be difficult to address. Conflicting views may be intense and divergent, but well-adjusted families have a healthy foundation for addressing them. The capability to resolve conflicts and solve problems gives family members confidence and restores hope.

Reactivated conflicts   Sometimes old conflicts appear to have been resolved in families. This may turn out to be an illusion. The conflicts may have been buried or avoided so successfully they were forgotten. Family members may be shocked and dismayed when they realize the new conflict they experience is an old conflict that has been reactivated by a new situation. *Reactivated* conflicts in the family tend to focus on issues of independence and dependence, acceptance and rejection, and sibling rivalries that had become more obscure (Siegler and Hyer 1984).

When adult children assume the responsibility of caring for a parent, they commonly assume roles that would have been naturally associated with the parent. The parent tends to be viewed as less capable in some areas of functioning, perhaps acting less like an adult. Alzheimer's disease affects adults in this manner. As children take care of their parent the roles are reversed. At times they may view the parent's behavior as childish. Some children view the parent as a child and treat him or her as they would a child, perhaps the way they remember being treated as children. Within the reactivated conflict, old feelings surface. Role reversals may reactivate conflicts experienced by families involved in the care of Alzheimer's disease victims.

Dependent needs change   An adult child, who had depended upon the parent affected by Alzheimer's disease, may resent the disease and the parent because his or her source of dependency is severely threatened. Continued demands of the parent will produce problems in coping with the illness for both the parent and the adult child. For the adult child, time to establish a more independent lifestyle is quickly running out. If the parent recognizes this, dealing with Alzheimer's disease is complicated by concerns for the welfare of the adult child. In cases where the dependent adult child is the primary source of support, there may be additional concerns about that individual's capacity to provide what will be needed. These family members are likely to become so bonded to one another, it may be difficult for other family members to effectively assist with the needed care.

The caregiver spouse may find it necessary to seek the assistance of children who have been rejected by the other parent. As these children become involved, the behavior of the parent—even though it may be influenced by brain damage and a disease process—may be looked upon as a manifestation of earlier rejection. At first, a child may refuse to help because it is awkward to manage the parent's behavior. The real reason may be related to feelings associated with an old conflict that has been reactivated.

The increased dependence of parents and resolution of old conflicts represents a *filial* crisis that faces all adult children (Margaret Blenkner 1983). In order for adult children to resolve the conflicts associated with this crisis, they must accept the dependencies of their parents. This involves clarifying the confusion associated with new roles that develop between children and their parents. Parents, from whom adult children had sought support in times of emotional trouble and economic pressure, now need the comfort and support of their children.

New views of parent   The acceptance of this role requires adult children to develop a vastly different view of the relationship they have with their parents. Through this view, children recognize and accept the interdependent future of parents without ignoring or invalidating their independent past (Eyde and Rich 1983). They "mature" into a role that is supportive of the potential for remaining independent and responsive to developing dependencies. This is superior to the idea of simple role reversal because it integrates the image of who parents "were" with who they "are." Alzheimer's disease changes what a parent can do. This threatens our view of who they were. Our responses to their needs must support their dignity and not ignore the memory of who they were. The mature child has resolved the conflicts of the "filial crisis" or refuses to allow them to interfere with his or her ability to respond positively and effectively to the needs of an afflicted parent.

Cohesive vs. Fragmented Families

Some families become closer during crises. Individual members are concerned about the views of other family members. Cohesive families function as a unit rather than isolated individuals. This provides a sense of belonging and a stronger impression that it is the family addressing a crisis, not separate individuals who cannot stick together. Even families that experience a good deal of conflict can prove to be cohesive (Blazer 1984). Families that are more fragmented are likely to experience more tension than cohesive families. This leaves them with less energy available to address the challenges posed by caregiving.

Relating to outside help   Professionals involved in Alzheimer's care will find it easier to develop alliances with more cohesive families. If your family is quite fragmented, professionals may encounter a "string" of different individuals. When the style of family interactions is also conflictual, professional alliances may be more difficult to maintain. A fragmented and conflictual family, over time, jeopardize the professional affiliations that would be supportive of the family's responses.

Productive vs. Nonproductive Families

Families who can work together in providing care are more likely to be productive. Families who cannot work together are less likely to be productive. Productivity is not simply a matter of "working together," since it involves the ability of families to plan, organize, and delegate responsibilities and activities. Some families have the potential to be productive, but if the person who had mobilized the family is stricken by Alzheimer's disease, new leadership needs to develop. Different types of family styles have different responses to this need. The fact that the spouse or daughter is most likely to become the primary provider of care also influences the development of new roles in the family.

Degree of involvement   Often it seems the primary caregiver is the only family member involved in the caregiving. They are unable or unwilling to involve other family members in some aspect of responding to the enormous demands they face. They are the only family member involved. In such cases, the potential productivity of the family's response to care is greatly reduced.

This may occur for several reasons. The involvement of some family members may increase conflict. A source of potential conflict is eliminated when these members are absent. Geographical or emotional distance between family members may separate them from the hands-on caregiving. There may be no other family members. In order to preserve their relationships with the victim of Alzheimer's, caregivers become extremely attached to the loved one. This emotional attachment may push other family members away. It is a source of frustration and reduced family productivity when other members could help and want to help.

Caregivers of persons with Alzheimer's disease must manage incredible stress. The daily care takes its toll on their physical, emotional, and mental resources. They are involved in a progressive, incomplete loss. The burdens of care pile up, and their productivity is threatened. Hope fades and caregivers resign themselves to what cannot be changed.

Fragile vs. Stable Families

The fragile versus stable characteristics of families affect the functioning of the family over time, not just at the moment of crisis. Since a family unit consists of individuals, the stability of those individuals must also be considered. Families who face Alzheimer's disease have faced crises before. It is helpful to examine the ways these crises were handled, and how the family was affected by them. For example, if a family member experienced a fairly significant health problem in the past, how supportive were other members of the family? Did they temporarily assume responsibilities or roles that had been associated with this individual? Were their expectations of recovery reasonable? Did the family unite to deal with the crisis or were they remarkably unconcerned?

Families facing Alzheimer's disease are not addressing problems and needs that can be quickly handled or easily dismissed. Caregiving will last a long time. Family members will be required to contend with unfamiliar and unpredictable situations. A stable family will be better prepared to address these situations over time; a fragile family will have greater difficulty providing sufficient support unless a healthier member assumes the primary role.

The members of a stable family are likely to be stable as individuals. If difficulties in relationships develop, they are resolved in reasonable ways without the family being disabled. The history of family relationships and interactions is not riddled with recurrent problems and long-standing conflicts. Support from children can be counted on because they are not continually absorbed by their emotional or relational problems.

Alzheimer's disease may develop in a family that has been characteristically stable, but as a result of the health problems, the stability of the family itself has been threatened. Alzheimer's is more likely to develop in older family members. Potentially supportive siblings and children may be older themselves. The spouse who becomes the caregiver may have chronic health problems that are magnified by stress and less attention to their own needs for care.

Energy drain   Tension is always seen in families that are fragile and fragmented. This reduces the energy available for being productive and may support the need for greater utilization of resources in the community. Families who have successfully met prior crises and maintained healthy interactions and productivity still have a good chance of meeting the caregiver's challenge if they can be flexible enough to involve other sources of support.

Family Roles and Rules

If the person affected by Alzheimer's disease had been the one who provided leadership and stability to the family, any type of family will experience the impact of his or her loss. Some families will be more adept than others in filling this gradually increasing void. Other family members must become available to assume this role or parts of it. They must be willing to accept the role, and the family must be open to this kind of change. Some families may have such rigid roles that other family members would be reluctant to assume the responsibilities. The roles within the family may be so unclear or mixed that the need for a designated leader might not at first be apparent.

Some families have very clear procedures or rules for responding to problems. A family hierarchy may exist that dictates in advance how changes in leadership should be handled. Even these may not sufficiently address how other family members assume new roles until the family comprehends what Alzheimer's does to the abilities of the affected person. The family's sensitivity to this person's remaining capabilities and wishes also influences how new roles of leadership are developed. Cultural differences also influence how rigid or flexible families can be in changing roles within the family.

Flexible responses   The presence of Alzheimer's disease in a family demands a family response. The flexibility of the family in responding to a situation that requires change in leadership is critical. Flexibility enables them to adapt and change, regroup and develop new patterns in any established hierarchy so that the family can care for the relative who is impaired (Blazer 1984). A family that is characterized by flexibility is less likely to be burdened by the weight of resigned or pessimistic attitudes.

Guides for relating   The quality of family interactions influences family communication and problem solving. It is also helpful to examine the factors in family relationships that influence the degree to which family members are involved with one another. Invisible boundaries exist in families. These boundaries act like rules that suggest how closely family members should be involved in each other's lives (Miller 1982). In some families, these boundaries are very clear so that interactions within the family are neither too involved nor too distant. Children have supportive alliances with each other, and the boundaries that characterize their involvement with parents are clear. The response of this type of family to the problems and needs created by Alzheimer's disease will be more readily defined. Issues concerning how involved each member is to become are not so confusing.

Disengaged families   There are other families where the boundaries influencing the usual degree of involvement result in too little or too much response. The degree of involvement tends to be consistent whether the family issues have major or minor significance. Disengaged families are at one extreme end of the continuum of involvement. Boundaries in these families are quite rigid. This rigidity inhibits communication. The elderly in this type of family are likely to be emotionally isolated from both their children and their siblings. If the diagnosis of Alzheimer's is made, the spouse is unlikely to request help from her family unless the level of her stress becomes quite extreme. Even in this situation, she would be hesitant to share many of her thoughts or feelings with her family (Miller 1982). Alzheimer's care in this family is likely to be a solitary activity. The likelihood of the caregiver to become overwhelmed would appear to be high unless other supportive resources are developed outside the home.

Enmeshed families   At the other extreme of the continuum of involvement, the enmeshed family is characterized as being so close its members lose their own sense of autonomy. Members of this family will have a very strong sense of belonging, but very low sense of their own ability in mastering skills, or appreciating the individually-determined abilities they may have acquired. Individuals in the enmeshed family are not given the opportunity to solve problems in their own way and own time, so it would have been difficult to learn and grow from any stressful experiences that preceded the crisis of Alzheimer's disease. The excessive concern and involvement characteristic of enmeshed families produces intense over-reactions, particularly during periods of stress (Miller 1982). What is stressful to these families may not be that stressful to other families. While the Alzheimer's victim in this family will have physical and other concrete needs met, these needs will be met at the expense of the victim's self-worth and individuality. Parents and children can be so overinvolved in each other's lives, that when one member is down or depressed, they all tend to suffer.

The overinvolvement that characterizes the enmeshed family can produce overload during Alzheimer's caregiving. As time passes, the energy for mutual support may have been expended on minor details so that the family as a whole has less to give. Fortunately, most families are not characteristically either enmeshed or disengaged. Styles that are more prominently enmeshed or disengaged may inhibit individuals providing Alzheimer's care; they need not prohibit it. When family problems persist that do interfere with care, professional help should be sought.

Family Roles During Crisis

Individuals in a family may take on different roles to cope with the situations and demands associated with Alzheimer's disease. Generally these roles are supportive of the impaired person and enable the family to cope adequately. Different roles may be assumed by different family members at various times. Several roles may be assumed by the same family member.

The Role of Facilitator

The stability of the family is the most important thing to the facilitator. Although other members of a family will support the involvement of a professional to determine what was wrong with a family member, the facilitator would have opposed this suggestion. This family member would probably obstruct other family efforts to get help for the impaired person, for example, getting second opinions or seeking psychiatric treatment for the psychiatric manifestations of the disease. They believe, consciously or unconsciously, that all members of the family, including themselves, are best served by keeping the relatives in a sick or more dependent role. Thus, they facilitate and encourage the illness and the problems associated with it. If the diagnosis has been made, the facilitator may oppose it being made known if they perceive it as a threat to the equilibrium of the family.

Other care-related decisions may involve additional family members in the facilitator role. The family stability may return once family members have had the chance to adjust and make the necessary changes in their lifestyles. Family members become more resistant to changes once things have settled down. They probably realize that changes in routine can be unsettling to everyone. If a support group member encourages a family member to explore adult day care or respite care, the suggestion might threaten the stability the family has achieved in its present response to a loved one's needs. The stress of the caregiver or the deteriorating status of the Alzheimer's victim are not considered. It is better to maintain the perceived stability of the family than upset this balance, as fragile as it might be.

The Role of Victim

The victim is the individual in the family who is most likely to have the most contact with other family members. He or she is quite likely to also have the most contact with professionals. There may be one or more victims in a family. Different family members at different times may assume the victim role. The victim views Alzheimer's as a direct and personal threat for a number of reasons. If they have been dependent upon the stricken individual, their own well-being, particularly in the future, might be at stake. Spouses may feel at risk since their relationship and marriage is threatened by the disease. Other family members are victims because their future with a loved one has been dramatically changed. The genetic fears of Alzheimer's families certainly contribute to the perception of the victim role. The frequency of family interactions may be reduced for all family members, but the caregiver spouse may also become isolated from friends. The disease threatens relationships. The victim would feel less threatened if someone could reverse the course Alzheimer's disease has taken. Professionals working with victims in a family may receive more criticism because they are unable to remove the ultimate personal threat, death.

The Role of Manager

When a family crisis occurs, one family member often takes charge. He or she is calm during the crisis and can be a stabilizing force.

Emotions are usually contained and this person may be somewhat intellectual in contacts with professionals. The explanations given to family members by the "manager" will be more intellectual than emotional in content. He may not be able to give as much emotional support, but plays a key role in organizing the family's response to what needs to be done. The family member can be an important liaison with professionals who become involved in caring for the needs of the affected family member and the primary family caregiver. The family manager is not usually as involved in the intimate aspects of care, and may maintain some distance from family members who are. Family members who live some distance from where the care is provided to love ones can assume some part of this family role. Their assistance with practical problem solving is supportive to an emotionally drained caregiver. Providing practical assistance supports the family manager's sense of being a part of the family's response to the disease.

The Role of Caretaker

Caretakers are those persons in the family who have an innate need to nurture the sick. They may have assumed this role in the family or chosen a profession that supports the fulfillment of this need. Many caretakers may be women who assume this role because of an innate need, or give in to social pressures that assign this role to them. Husbands are thought to suffer less stress as Alzheimer's caregivers because it gives them the opportunity to reciprocate in kind to wives who nurtured them and their children.

The caregivers' need to nurture may obscure their need to care for themselves. When they view their relative as a helpless child, there is a good chance their nurturing tendencies will recreate a relationship with the spouse or parent that resembles the relationship they would have with a child. This reinforces a rebonding process that may lead to an inseparable bond. The relationship becomes resistant to any threat of separation. Caretakers frequently avoid any opportunities for respite. As a result, they frequently wear themselves out to the point they have no desire for any useful or meaningful activity. Their life is singularly consumed by caring for a loved one. Any other family attempt to separate them from this consuming activity will be resisted because it is "all they can do" for the loved one.

The caretaker role may be motivated by guilt. It is a role that corresponds to the overinvolvement stage of grief during family adjustment. Caretakers may remain "stuck" at this stage because the role itself seems to encourage overinvolvement. When the Alzheimer's patient dies, the person who has become entrenched in the caretaker role can suffer a tremendous void. They have not only lost a loved one, they have lost a role that sustained them. Caretakers may experience a severe and prolonged grief reaction.

Escapee

Escapees may be found in many types of families, but they are more frequently found in families characterized by intense conflict. Some escapees may have left severely enmeshed families in order to find autonomy as worthwhile individuals. The escapee has withdrawn from the usual interactions in the family. They are often blamed for not showing up in the Alzheimer's crisis. They are criticized for failing to show more concern or providing more care.

Absence protects   It is not unusual for the escapee to have moved some distance from the family and become involved in activities that are more rewarding and appreciative of them as worthwhile persons. They try to compensate for past relationships and interactions that had been unhealthy. Their withdrawal from their families is self-protective. While they may function well outside of their family, they seem to realize they cannot tolerate re-involvement in a highly stressed and conflictual family (Blazer 1984), even if a parent is dying with Alzheimer's disease. They would rather leave the terrible business of the past unfinished. Their absence may be quite acceptable to some family members. However, the parent who becomes the caregiver might wish that old matters could be put aside to allow the family to be together during a time of crisis.

The Role of Patient

The person with Alzheimer's disease is the patient. He or she has the problem that clearly precipitated the crisis for the family. This problem then creates further stresses on the emotional, physical, mental, spiritual, and financial resources available to the family as a whole. As the patient, the Alzheimer's victim will be the focus of these resources. However, other family members may assume the role of a "hidden patient" when they seek professional help for a loved one. They use their relationship and helping role with the patient to get their own needs addressed. Contact with professional also affords them the opportunity to bring up old issues and problems. These problems may not be directly related to Alzheimer's disease but influence the ability of family members to provide care, support one another, and generally participate in caregiving. Some issues may directly relate to family issues that still affect their capability to work together productively.

Hidden patient   The needs of these family members seem to be in competition with the relative who has Alzheimer's disease. They have legitimate needs that warrant professional attention. Uncomfortable in seeking help directly for themselves, they seize the opportunity on the coattails of the relative. No other disease has given so much credence to the idea that the needs of caregivers are as legitimate as the needs of the person identified as the patient. Unfortunately, family members who are caretakers may not be able to balance meeting their needs and the needs of loved ones. They should consider professional help. The needs of the caregiver and patient must be addressed with more balanced responses from the professionals and health care system.

Caregivers and Caregiving

The need to care for people who are vulnerable, or needy in some way, is a strong social value. Some people make a profession of taking care of people who have problems and needs of one kind or another. Some caregivers are strongly motivated by the need to nurture, but not all caregivers are "caretakers." Different approaches to caregiving can be influenced by the roles just discussed. Since caregiving occurs within a family and a relationship, these relational factors further characterize the process. What we call *caregiving* involves an attitude of caring and the expression of this attitude through actions. In such cases, professionals must quickly recognize that the needs of caregivers are as significant as the patients.

Taking care of people we love can be viewed as an obligation or expectation of families. As much as 80 percent of the care elderly persons receive is provided by family members who become caregivers. But it is more difficult to care for members of our families if our motivation is solely a sense of duty or obligation. Resentment and similar feelings breed more readily when care is performed out of a sense of family obligation. There must be other reasons for caring.

Several years ago I had the opportunity to speak at two consecutive conferences, one in El Paso and another in Baltimore. Both were sponsored by the Alzheimer's organization in those cities. At that time, the sponsors were extremely concerned about the difficulties support groups had in reaching many of the family caregivers who had become isolated and overinvolved. They were equally concerned in reaching caregivers who had become so overwhelmed their physical and mental health had been jeopardized. Offers of help had been rejected, and these caregivers continued along a path that would surely lead to greater risks for themselves and their loved ones. By this time, there were a number of very helpful books available to caregivers. Social research had inundated journals with studies concerning caregiver stresses, strains and burdens. Although very little research had addressed how "persons" with the disease coped, research had begun to look more carefully at how "caregivers" coped with stress. The impact of grief on caregivers and loved ones losing themselves to a disease was beginning to receive more attention.

In one sense, caregiving was a job. A job description would be appropriate to introduce caregivers to the job they had accepted. In some cases, it had been accepted out of choice; in other cases, there may not have been a choice. It needed to be done. And despite the fact most family caregivers did not have the prerequisite skills, they had performed the job as well as anyone. It had been difficult, but they learned to manage strange behaviors, adjust to a more rigid routine and solve problems without the benefit of reasoning. Some had even learned a few things that would benefit nurses, psychiatrists, and neurologists. Others had acquired a rudimentary knowledge of family law. Some were proud of the fact they had learned to do the things their spouses had claimed they would never be able to do. Let's look back at the job description more closely.

Caregivers work with virtually no supervision. They are their own supervisors with a staff of one who has some trouble performing his or her job according to expectations. Fortunately, this job does not require one to sleep although at times the sole staff person who needs to sleep doesn't, especially when it would be beneficial. For a job that is performed without a salary, one could at least expect some type of benefits. A few days off would be a good start. A good physical or a mental health day sure wouldn't hurt. Unfortunately, the benefits look suspiciously like a plan for growth and development. For example, any decent job should increase your self-esteem. This one expects you to accept your life and recognize how it is still meaningful. Worst of all, it would be disgraceful to quit even if you didn't like the job. When you accept the job, things are a little confusing. Come to think of it, there was something else mentioned in the job description about confusion. But it is clearer now what "risk of isolation" means. And the warnings about the job creating high levels of stress are not exaggerated.

Becoming a caregiver is a little like starting a new job. At least you know the person you work for, and you have known them for a long time. Much of what you know about them is still helpful. Like other bosses, they give you more feedback about your performance when you first start than later when you might need it more. When you do something wrong these bosses are more likely to act differently rather than tell you what you need to change. Other family members act like they are in the workplace. They are not really your supervisor but they always know what you should do.

More than a job
Becoming a caregiver involves much more than performing job duties, because what you do happens within an established relationship that is one among many others in a family. Caregiving is not really a role but it refers to the care that is given within established roles like husband-wife, parent-child (Pearlin et al. 1990). When this care is given out of affection, it is more positively meaningful than similar actions resulting from a sense of duty and obligation.

Caring involves feelings

Caring is the part of our commitment to the welfare of other persons that involves our feelings about them and our emotional reactions to experiences involving them. Caregiving is the "behavioral" expression of this commitment (Pearlin et al. 1990). Giving care to a parent, spouse, or sibling is an extension of caring about that person. Both caring and caregiving are present in all relationships where people attempt to protect and enhance each other's well-being. When family members become caregivers, their commitments require they do something different for the person who needs their care. This alone does not change the fact they care. The experiences involved in caregiving will be new, and these may produce emotional reactions that are different in kind or intensity from those produced by previous experiences.

Alzheimer's disease inevitably leads to greater impairment. The progressively increasing dependency resulting from this impairment demands more caregiving activity. This, in turn, leads to profound changes in the relationship in which caregiving occurs. The give and take in the relationship had flowed back and forth. As the needs and dependencies of relatives become greater, the "give" flows in one direction. Caregiving may expand to the point it occupies virtually the whole relationship. This means that the affection that was originally associated with caring flows but does not come back. Ultimately, a cherished relationship comprised of two people is transformed into one in which one person is caregiving for the other. This dramatic and involuntary transformation is itself a major source of stress.

Caring for caregiver

Family caregivers directly face this transformation of a relationship. Other family members experience it as well, but are not confronted by it daily. The caring part of the family caregiver receives less and less encouragement from the loved one to whom he or she gives care. As concerned as family members and friends may be about the relative who is being transformed by Alzheimer's disease, their concern about the relative who is the caregiver may seem greater. Their concerns may be interpreted as comments about the quality of caregiving, even though these messages are really about caring. Their behavior is their own attempt "to be" a caregiver "for" a caregiver. They may be attempting to increase the diminishing flow of assistance and affection.

Caring about caregiving   Sometimes the attempts of other family members to give to the caregiver are frustrated, and the caregiver believes these same family members may "not" care. When you are losing a relationship and a person, you do not stop giving care. The part of you that is caring may need to be nurtured, but your expression of "caring" seems to be reduced to "caregiving." Your reactions to the experience of caregiving begin to involve feelings that are inconsistent with the caring part of you. Anger toward your loved one leads to guilt. You may wish the caregiving would end, but that would mean the relationship would end. It would be nice to have help and take a break, but what if something happened while you were gone. You have needs, too. You feel drained and empty, but what are these feelings when they are compared to what your loved one feels? Whenever caregivers begin to respond to their own needs, they are reminded of the conflicts that seem to be inherent in caring simultaneously for two persons. It is always easier to give into the voice that says the other's needs are greater when you are too tired to be sure anymore.

Providing for the needs of two people was not as difficult when both people could speak for themselves. You knew each other well enough to know the preferences of the other. But in time, the other person can no longer speak for himself. Then it becomes questionable whether preferences make that much difference. Alzheimer's— must it change everything? How can I separate myself from its grip? How can I feel that I am part of a family again? How do I know when it is O.K. to be myself in other ways again? When am I no longer just a caregiver?

Care for self   Caregivers reach a point where it is important to them to be whole individuals again. They want more of life, even in the face of the losses they endure. Some recognize this after the mourning becomes less intense and they decide to go on living. Some do grow and develop during this experience. But the social and personal injunctions to care are very powerful. Caregivers need something to guide them in making choices that help them care for themselves. They need something that suggests it is their moral and ethical right to consider their own needs. They need something to empower them to take care of themselves. Participation in Alzheimer's family support groups is supportive because caregivers see "their" dilemmas are the same for virtually "all" caregivers. These support groups often develope a Caregivers' Bill of Rights (Gwyther 1990).

The idea of a formalized Bill of Rights is healthy. It provides some balance to offset the moral and social injunctions caregivers sense from society, family, and their respective cultures. It also asserts that individuals and families are more important than the unrelenting tasks of caregiving itself—even when those tasks are an expression of caring. The idea of sacrificing our lives for another may be viewed as heroic and noble, when we are fully conscious of what we are doing. Otherwise, it is self-destructive and unnecessary. Caregivers do not willingly embrace this idea of sacrificing their lives.

The sample Caregivers' Bill of Rights that follows can help caregivers find the balance that supports their value, and the value of those for whom they care. It also encourages caregivers to exercise these rights for the sake of their health and the health of loved ones. Some of these loved ones are victims of Alzheimer's disease. Others are family members with whom relationships will still exist when caregiving has ended.

These rights apply to the life of the family as aptly as they do to the life of the family caregiver. For many caregivers, learning to become a part of their families again is as worthy a goal as establishing their own separate identities once caregiving has ended and the presence of grief has become more pronounced.

Caregivers' Bill of Rights

In as much as WE, THE CAREGIVERS, devote both ourselves and our resources to the care, maintenance and support of loved ones with Alzheimer's disease, we affirm that we have basic and inalienable rights.

We affirm that we are not alone in the challenge to maintain a dignified and humane lifestyle for ourselves and the loved ones for whom we care. Furthermore, we recognize that we are not alone in seeking better ways to accomplish this goal for loved ones and ourselves, and respect those who join us in this endeavor. As a result of the responsibility we knowingly accept for our loved ones, we must also accept responsibility for ourselves. Because of this we declare the following individual rights:

- The right to make decisions on behalf of loved ones and ourselves that support what is best for both of us.
- The right to have time and activities for ourselves without guilt, fear, or criticism.
- The right to have feelings that are inherently a part of losing someone we love.
- The right to deal with what we can alone, and the right to ask about what we do not understand.
- The right to seek options that reasonably accommodate our needs and the needs of our loved ones.
- The right to be treated with respect by those from whom we seek advice and assistance; the right to expect our loved ones to be treated in the same manner.
- The right to make mistakes and be forgiven.
- The right to be accepted as a vital and valued member of our families even when our views are different.
- The right to love ourselves and accept that we have done what was humanly possible.
- The right to learn what we can do and the time to learn it.
- The right to say goodbye before we must finally let go of the one we love.
- The right to be free from feelings and thoughts that are negative, destructive, and unfounded; and to work through feelings that are hard to understand.
- The right to develop our lives again before our endeavor of love is complete.

10

VALUES, BELIEFS, AND THE CAREGIVER EXPERIENCE

Expectations influence our feelings and reactions.

It is not an easy job to change our expectations or image of a person we have known for years. However, an examination of our beliefs about the Alzheimer victim's behavior can give caregivers new insights into interacting with loved ones. Using this revised perspective, the caregiver can gain more control of the situation and can help the person with Alzheimer's to retain his capacity to reason, understand, and act appropriately as long as possible.

Taking forgetfulness personally

What the caregiver believes about the Alzheimer's victim and behavior definitely influences what he feels and how he reacts. If he believes the loved one is asking the same questions over and over just to annoy him and thus becomes irritated, this irritation will be obvious to the Alzheimer's victim, even though he probably will not understand what he has done to annoy the caregiver. Such needless irritation is stressful for the caregiver, and it can have an emotionally unsettling effect on the Alzheimer's victim, leading to other, more complicated problems. It is therefore important that each caregiver learns not to take the victim's behavior personally.

Unrealistic expectations can lead to anger and frustration.

A caregiver's expectations of himself also affect how he cares for a loved one. Many caregivers put great pressure on themselves. Lacking a full understanding of the physical causes of the illness and its impact on the victim's functional capabilities, they hold themselves responsible for their relative's problems and failures. Anger, guilt, frustration, and similar feelings push the caregiver beyond his limits. Caregivers must realistically assess their limitations plus the resources available. Otherwise, the stress of caregiving can lead to desperation and fatigue.

Previous adjustments to illness and loss can predict our adjustment to Alzheimer's.

Caregivers must learn to solicit and accept the help of others during the course of the illness. Those of us who find this difficult should examine our beliefs. Do we believe it is our sole responsibility to provide for all the person's needs, or is it a responsibility to be shared by other family members? Also to be considered is how well we tend to take care of ourselves. In the past, have we become so consumed by the needs of our family and others that we neglected our own needs? In the caregiving role, how are we responding to the needs of our loved one? What beliefs do we have about our role? These questions are critical to the basic pattern of our caregiving.

The caregiver should allow the patient to remain as independent as possible.

As the disease progresses, the caregiver will find himself shouldering increased responsibility for the patient. In particular, a child may find himself caring for a parent with Alzheimer's in ways that the parent once cared for him. This phenomenon is known as role reversal. It is very important, however, not to speed up this reversal process any sooner than is absolutely necessary. Alzheimer's disease is a gradually progressive illness, which means that a person does not lose all capabilities suddenly and simultaneously, nor does his family need to take over his total care all at once. The caregiver can best help the Alzheimer's patient by allowing him to remain as independent as possible for as long as possible. When the person providing care attempts to take control over all areas of the person's life simultaneously, some very unfortunate consequences such as the following may result.

- The person refuses to admit he needs any help at all and rejects all aid.
- The adult relationship between the caregiver and the afflicted person is severed prematurely.

- The self-concept of the Alzheimer's victim is eroded by doubts about his existing abilities.

- The person with Alzheimer's becomes prematurely dependent.

- The caregiver becomes overwhelmed by the unnecessary burden created.

Caregivers must therefore monitor themselves to make sure that, in their desire to be helpful, they do not hasten the end of the loved one's self-sufficient life.

Changes are not always obvious. On the other hand, family members may overlook symptoms of the disease and therefore fail to provide aid soon enough. If contact with the person is only occasional, they may have no reason to suspect that a medical condition is responsible for subtle changes in the person's grooming, dress, speech, or behavior.

It is normal to minimize changes in a loved one. When changes occur, particularly in a spouse, we tend to ignore them, if possible, or to attribute changes to temporary circumstances. It is often easier to dismiss things that irritate or bother us than it is to deal with them, especially when they do not seem to be cause for alarm. If the spouse continues to have problems, we may still feel hesitant to get a professional opinion.

Each member of the family adjusts differently. If the severity of the problems is more apparent to some family members than to others, conflict may arise among them about the best course of action. For example, Betty may want to play down her husband John's increasing problems with memory and suspicious ideas. When her son and daughter insist that she take their father to a doctor, Betty may deny that a problem exists, leading her son and daughter to become as distressed by their mother's behavior as by their father's. Betty is in conflict; her denial suggests she is having trouble thinking about the frightening possibilities. Additionally, there is the issue of convincing John to see a professional about problems he blames on her and others. Betty may believe that the family holds her responsible for what her husband is doing and what might be happening to him.

Examining beliefs helps caregivers respond more constructively to problems.   It is natural at times to have counterproductive reactions to the problems of Alzheimer's disease. It can be a very difficult balancing act to determine what caregivers can and cannot expect, how much assistance should be offered, and how much is too much. The point is that caregivers should not blame themselves or their loved one, but examine how their beliefs influence their thinking, the way they act and react, and the emotions they experience and express. Such a self-examination will help caregivers to respond more constructively as they begin to care for a family member who is affected by a disease that significantly changes his behavior and character before it changes his health.

A case study shows how beliefs influence actions.   The following personalized example will help to illustrate how a caregiver's beliefs can influence his reactions to a typical problem arising from a spouse's Alzheimer's condition.

Problem: Helen is yelling at her husband Tom. From the bedroom she screams, "Come here! You never come fast enough when I need you!" Then she bursts into tears.

Belief: Tom believes that his wife Helen depends on him too much and should do more for herself. He knows she has Alzheimer's, but he feels she is being lazy. He has always felt she was a demanding person. When he hears her crying, he thinks to himself that it is just like her to get hysterical about nothing.

What beliefs relate to Tom's thoughts and feelings?   Because he thinks Helen is just being lazy, Tom feels aggravated. This feeling grows as he considers how often she depends on him to do things that she really could do for herself. He is already washing dishes, which is not his job. Her crying irritates him more than it frightens or concerns him; he believes she cries to get what she wants. Because he feels manipulated, he becomes angrier.

Tom's reaction: "Helen, shut up! I'll be there in a minute, or you can come in here." Tom is too angry to ask her what she needs or to go to the bedroom immediately. He disregards the fact that his wife now has difficulties in clearly expressing her needs.

Helen's problem: Actually, Helen has slipped out of the chair in her bedroom. She is not hurt, but she is frightened and upset. She has made statements in the past about her husband not coming to her when she asked, even before the Alzheimer's condition, and that almost habitual response has slipped out when, in a panic, she cannot describe what has really happened. The disease has affected her coordination, and in her fright, she cannot organize her movements to pull herself up. She is crying out of fear and frustration.

Tom is reluctant to respond to the initial yelling because of past experiences. He still does not understand the impact of the illness well enough to appreciate how it is eroding his wife's ability to manage for herself. Neither does he appreciate the insecurity created by the illness.

With a clearer understanding of Helen's limitations, Tom might ask her if something is wrong or simply walk into the bedroom. He has probably gotten tired of taking care of his wife and feels frustration and anger. These negative reactions toward his wife are intensified by his feelings of being unappreciated. His irritation has delayed his response to Helen, who is sitting on the floor unable to get up, feeling frightened and upset.

Caregivers can respond more appropriately to problems when they identify the various reasons for their reactions. The previous illustration shows that the perceived problem is not always the real problem, and that beliefs and feelings about a problem can lead to interpretations, judgments, and reactions which can prevent caregivers from successfully handling the problem.

11

HOW TO RESPOND POSITIVELY TO ALZHEIMER'S BEHAVIORS

In Chapter 2, we discussed the symptoms of Alzheimer's disease. Even when we recognize a disturbing behavior on the part of our loved one as an Alzheimer's symptom, however, it is not always easy to know what the appropriate response should be. Unaccustomed to our loved one's new impairment, we naturally tend to respond to the behavior as we would have in the past when the person was healthy. Unfortunately, this often means responding with annoyance, frustration, and anger—which, as we have seen, is not helpful either for us or the Alzheimer's victim.

This chapter suggests more productive ways to respond to common disturbing behaviors exhibited by Alzheimer's patients. After listing the behavior, we first identify the common immediate reactions. Usually this is an interpretation and response that would be appropriate if we were responding to a healthy person's behavior, but it is not a useful response to behavior by an Alzheimer's patient. We then guide the reader through a better interpretation of the behavior, one based on an understanding of the brain impairment produced by Alzheimer's disease. Finally, we offer specific suggestions for productive ways of responding to the problem.

Our goal is to create an accurate and practical guide to caring for Alzheimer's patients that will help both caregivers and patients enjoy the good days and minimize the bad days. Our examples cannot possibly cover all situations. However, when caregivers learn this approach, they can use it with different situations and in different care settings.

Behavior	*1. The person asks the same questions over and over.*
Common Responses	The person is not listening or trying to remember; she wants attention or is trying to annoy you; she should be able to control this.
Alzheimer's Interpretation	The person is suffering memory loss, which in turn creates a strong sense of insecurity and uncertainty. She may be asking the same questions repeatedly because she seeks reassurance and

security, or perhaps your earlier answers seemed vague or unclear. She may sense you are avoiding the answer, which could heighten her sense of insecurity.

In more advanced stages, memory impairment may be so severe that she does not recall asking the question, or she may feel threatened by your earlier answer. For example, if she asks repeatedly when she is going to the doctor, the doctor may be a source of insecurity for her.

Helpful Responses

- Respond clearly, slowly, and concretely to questions.
- Have the person repeat what you have said.
- If you suspect that your earlier answer disturbed the person, provide reassurance and/or factual information that will set her mind at rest.
- Distract the person into other activity or other topics of discussion and ignore further questions.
- Avoid arguing or responding with anger; do not rebuke the person for the memory problem.
- Write down the information in question for the person who can still read.

Behavior	*2. The person's personality appears to have changed.*

Common Responses

He is going crazy or having a nervous breakdown; he has lost all self-respect and pride.

Alzheimer's Interpretation

Personality changes are characteristic symptoms of Alzheimer's. Often, these changes are observed prior to any clear impairment of memory or intellectual abilities. Brain impairment associated with Alzheimer's can radically change the way the person acts. Additionally, personality characteristics can be exaggerated in early phases of the illness.

Subtle changes in personality can represent an early signal that a problem exists. If the person realizes that he is acting in ways which are not like him, he may fear that he is having a nervous breakdown or losing his mind.

Eventually the brain impairment erases most traits of individuality. Some examples of personality changes follow:

Normal Personality	*New Traits*
Socially active	Socially withdrawn
Calm, easygoing	Worried, easily upset
Kind, understanding	Selfish, demanding
Relaxed	Paranoid
Emotionally controlled	Excessively emotional
Careful, cautious	Careless
Good judgment	Poor judgment
Sexually sensitive	Sexually demanding
Friendly	Unfriendly, hostile
Honest	Dishonest
Flexible	Rigid
Loving	Uncaring

Helpful Responses

- Accept personality changes as results of, or reactions to, brain impairment.
- Try to satisfy the needs underlying behavior, such as the person's need for security, self-esteem, dignity, and love.

Behavior	**3. The person does not do what she says she will or leaves a task uncompleted.**
Common Responses	She is lazy and not really trying; she is lying to you; she wants your help with everything.
Alzheimer's Interpretation	Memory impairment makes it more difficult to do something that was agreed upon. For example, seeing a shirt laid on the bed may no longer trigger the idea that the person should put it on.

Memory abilities cannot be separated from intellectual abilities, such as reasoning, and both faculties are being lost.

Helpful Responses

- Use reminders and memory lists.
- Maintain a routine for daily activities.
- Make requests close to the time the task is to be completed.
- Provide step-by-step assistance for more complicated tasks.
- Always request the desired behavior in the same setting (e.g. eating in kitchen or dining room, dressing in bedroom or bathroom).
- Provide verbal assistance if the person seems to have forgotten how to complete parts of the task or has forgotten what she is doing.

Behavior	**4. The person denies his memory problems and makes excuses for mistakes, blames others, or seems unaware of the problem.**
Common Responses	The person is not being honest; he should face the problem and accept responsibility for his own mistakes; he is just getting old and senile.
Alzheimer's Interpretation	Denial of memory problems is a very common response to Alzheimer's. Initially, denial is a necessary defense. It protects the person from

frightening changes that are difficult to accept. If he makes excuses or blames others, he may be desperately trying to explain the memory impairment without directly confronting the problem.

**Helpful
Responses**

- Avoid forcing the person to face up to the memory problems.
- Provide reminders or suggest checklists as ways to aid memory.
- Be understanding of the threat that memory impairment poses for your relative.
- Arrange for the person to talk to a professional if he seems troubled but cannot admit the problem to his family.

Behavior	*5. The person insists she does not need help because she has always done things for herself; she becomes angry when you offer assistance.*
Common Responses	She is stubborn and unreasonable; she is rejecting you personally; her anger is unfair.
Alzheimer's Interpretation	The person's refusal of help is an effort to maintain independence. Anger directed toward you may really be caused by her frustration with the illness. Her self-worth and self-esteem are threat-

ened. Later, such denial may show she has lost a grasp of her own needs and problems.

**Helpful
Responses**

- Determine what help is needed and provide what is needed in a kind manner.
- Realize that the person may genuinely lack awareness of her needs and problems.
- Provide encouragement and reinforcement for even the smallest successes and for acceptance of your help.
- Avoid overemphasizing the person's weaknesses or communicating disgust.

- Avoid confronting problems too directly if you suspect the confrontation could provoke strong emotional reactions.

Behavior	*6. A spouse's sexual interests and demands are higher than normal or more difficult for you to satisfy.*
Common Responses	A sexual relationship is inappropriate in light of the illness. How could he enjoy sexual activity at such a time?
Alzheimer's Interpretation	Brain damage can increase a person's desire for sexual activity. It also can decrease his sexual inhibitions, create difficulties in relating sexually, and reduce sensitivity to his partner. Alzheimer's

can threaten a person's sexual identity and self-esteem.

The loss of intimacy that occurs as the disease gradually diminishes the victim's personality may make it difficult for the caregiver to sustain a sexual relationship. The affected person may continue to find sexual satisfaction, but the spouse suffers a loss of emotional satisfaction.

Despite these problems, sexual relations can continue to be important, and they are a matter of personal choice. The person with Alzheimer's needs to feel wanted and loved. Adjustments in relating sexually may be necessary.

Helpful Responses

- Understand changing sexual interests and demands in the context of both the illness and your prior sexual relationship.
- Rely upon touching, being caressed, and nonverbal relating as substitutes for the sex act.
- Talk with a physician or counselor if the sexual problems persist.

Behavior	*7. The person mishandles her money and monthly bills; she accuses you and others of stealing her*

money; she claims her banker is handling money matters.

Common Responses	She is inconsiderate and irresponsible; she is unfair and will not face the facts; she is lying and avoiding the issue.
Alzheimer's Interpretation	Having and handling money is one of the symbols of a person's independence and competence. The person may blame others for her mistakes because she is trying to protect her self-esteem

and maintain her independence.

Early problems with memory and reasoning abilities make it difficult to handle more complex financial matters. Trying to perform calculations, even on paper, becomes frustrating. Accusing others of taking money is one way in which the person fills the gaps in her memory and protects her self-esteem.

Helpful Responses

- Be sure there is no truth to accusations of theft, particularly when the person lives alone and is vulnerable.

- Let the spouse or adult child assume the responsibility for financial matters.

- Monitor the person's monthly bills and contact creditors about questionable charges.

- Be sensitive to the person's insecurity and fears when discussing financial matters.

- Allow the person to have some cash on hand to enable an easier adjustment to alternative financial arrangements.

- Consider legal arrangements such as power of attorney and guardianship as means of protecting the person's financial security.

Behavior	*8. The person tells ridiculous stories or says unusual things.*

Common Responses	He is lying or being mean; he is going crazy or getting senile.
Alzheimer's Interpretation	Such stories are easy to take personally, but they are rarely malicious. As memory and reasoning abilities continue to decline, larger gaps are left in the person's perception of reality. It is harder for

him to explain or understand what is happening because his grasp of logic is deteriorating. Ridiculous stories and obvious untruths may be attempts to fill in the blanks, to explain what he cannot understand.

If the person believes his own stories, the things he says may cause real agitation, anger, and fearfulness. If his stories place blame on others, he may be trying to defend his self-respect and integrity.

Some of the unusual things a person says may also represent difficulties in speech. Finding words to explain things or even name things correctly becomes difficult as the disease develops. The person may be able to manage only fragmentary ideas or statements.

Helpful Responses

- Clarify and correct the person's understanding of events.
- Respond sensitively to underlying feelings of insecurity, fear, or frustration.
- Avoid overreacting to stories or allowing an argument to start.
- Distract the person with conversation about other things.
- If the person is upset, give him a chance to calm down.

Behavior	*9. The person wants things to be done immediately; she wants you to do everything.*
Common Responses	The person is being inconsiderate; she is acting childish and overly dependent; she is attempting to control you.
Alzheimer's Interpretation	If the person was demanding before the brain impairment, the disease could accentuate such traits. In addition, her loss of memory may have

triggered anxiety and panic, and her demanding or overly dependent behavior may be an attempt to gain control. Her anger may mask fear.

**Helpful
Responses**

- Remind yourself that there is no point in becoming frustrated and angry.
- Respond calmly.
- Let the person know what is going on and being done.
- Do something with the person, even if not what is being asked.
- Talk to other people about your feelings, frustrations.

Behavior	**10. The person repeatedly talks about experiences from the past.**
Common Responses	He is living in the past; he does not want to relate to the present.
Alzheimer's Interpretation	Although the brain-impaired person's ability to recall recent experiences is becoming less reliable, he still may remember more remote material from the past. This material remains ac-

cessible to the person longer and can provide a more meaningful basis for self-esteem and identity. The present has become more threatening and difficult to accept emotionally. The person may also be losing his ability to relate to time and may be confused about the relation of past to present.

**Helpful
Responses**

- Use past memories to make activities in the present more meaningful.
- Provide concrete information that distinguishes the present from the past; for example, contrast pictures of grown-up grandchildren with their childhood pictures.

- Set aside time for reminiscing.
- Patiently and supportively orient the person to the present when confusion is apparent.

Behavior	*11. The person's abilities fluctuate from day to day or hour to hour; she remembers some things but not others.*
Common Responses	She remembers what she wants to; she is not trying to remember; she must be getting old and senile.
Alzheimer's Interpretation	It is normal for the memory of all Alzheimer's patients to fluctuate in this fashion. It is a mistake to believe that improved memory on a given day means the condition is improving, however.

Some information or events may be easier to remember. Material that is unpleasant or threatening may be more easily forgotten.

Helpful Responses

- Make the most of good days.
- Determine the kinds of information more easily recalled.
- Note if a certain manner of presenting information improves some kinds of memory.
- Realize that the person will tend to remember more under relaxed and quiet circumstances.

Behavior	*12. The person continues to drive the car despite safety problems.*
Common Responses	He is being stubborn and showing poor judgment; he should give up driving.
Alzheimer's Interpretation	Driving gives a person freedom and control of his daily life. Denying he is lost or confused, despite

obvious problems, is his way of defending her self-esteem and independence. Confronting him about mistakes may produce more vigorous denial and angry reactions.

Despite resistance, family members must limit and eventually eliminate the person's driving opportunities. Even during the early stages of the illness, the person is vulnerable in situations requiring quick decisions because his reaction time is impaired. Alzheimer's also affects visual perception, including perception of distance.

Concentration difficulties will eventually erode the person's ability to drive safely. For example, if the traffic light before him changes to green but a car on the intersecting street is going through the red light, the brain-impaired person may be unable to decide which change is the most important. Too many things are happening at once, and his problem-solving abilities become overwhelmed.

Giving up driving is very difficult for most people with Alzheimer's. They may be more willing to stop driving if another health problem, such as visual impairment, is cited as the reason. Most caregivers will want a loved one to stop driving long before the affected person is ready.

Helpful Responses

- Enlist the support of other family members in convincing the person to stop driving.
- Enlist the help of the person's physician, attorney, insurance agent, mental health professional, or trusted friend; the instructions of authority figures may be followed more closely.
- Discuss the problem with your insurance representative.
- Contact your police department or department of public safety and inquire about license nonrenewal, suspension, or restrictions and other procedures to ground an unsafe driver.
- Remove keys or dismantle the car's starter as a last resort.
- Understand the person's anger and resentment about such a loss and avoid confrontations about driving difficulties.
- Remember that removal of driving responsibilities eliminates the possibility of an unfortunate accident.

Behavior	*13. The person accuses you, family, and friends of doing things or makes up stories about you.*
Common Responses	She is becoming paranoid, losing her mind, being unfair, becoming unmanageable, or trying to hurt or embarrass you; she is getting senile.
Alzheimer's Interpretation	Such problems are other ways in which brain-impaired persons react to the insecurity created by memory loss. In this case, the problem more directly involves the caregiver, since the victim is

most likely to accuse her spouse and other close family members.

Arguments tend to reinforce beliefs. Confrontations and other negative approaches tend to worsen the situation rather than help it.

Helpful Responses

- Avoid contradicting the person directly, as this may only make her angry and confused.
- Avoid highlighting mistakes and give calm and reasonable explanations; communicate a sense that things are all right or will improve.
- If something is lost, offer to help find it or suggest specific places it could be found.

Behavior	*14. The person has hallucinations or bizarre and frightening delusions.*
Common Responses	The person is mentally ill; Alzheimer's is getting worse.
Alzheimer's Interpretation	Progressive brain impairment affects an individual's ability to interpret information accurately. Hallucinations are often misinterpretations of real sights and sounds. Delusional beliefs repre-

sent an attempt to fill in gaps of information and explain what happened. For example, if the person says someone is knocking on the walls and is trying to break into his house, he may really have heard a tree branch rubbing against the house. Insecurity, so often associated with progressive brain impairment, leads the person to interpret events from a fearful and threatening perspective. Suspiciousness is a common response to a person's diminishing control of her world.

When a person seems to be talking with someone who is not present, he may not actually see or hear the person, but he may be involved in a delusional belief, such as thinking a deceased person is alive or talking to a child who lives 400 miles away.

A number of other problems contribute to hallucinations and delusional beliefs. These include medical problems such as infections, changes in diabetic conditions, or pernicious anemia. Medications also must be evaluated.

Other conditions that impair a person's ability to receive information can contribute to hallucinations or delusional beliefs. Hearing or visual impairment are examples.

**Helpful
Responses**

- When delusions or hallucinations are observed, consult a physician.
- Provide the person with concrete information.
- Show support for the feeling of the experience, responding with reassurance.
- Avoid arguing or disagreeing with the person, as that will only upset him more.
- Try to distract the person, move him to another room, or talk about something comforting.

Behavior	*15. The person becomes disinterested and withdrawn in social situations.*
Common Responses	She does not care about friends or people anymore; she wants you to stay home all the time.
Alzheimer's Interpretation	The person's cognitive and memory deficits are making it very difficult to follow social conversations and interact appropriately. This inability

leads to frustration and anxiety in social situations, thus prompting her to withdraw.

This withdrawal may be preceded by restlessness, tension, and agitation. If the demands on the person are not decreased, she may become more upset or even rude to uninformed observers.

**Helpful
Responses**

- Provide emotional support and verbal assistance in demanding social situations and observe any obvious changes in the person's anxiety level.

- When the person becomes nervous, encourage her to simply withdraw from the social situation for a while.

- Anticipate the more demanding situations before they become uncomfortable.

- Inform friends about her behavior and how they can make her participation easier.

- Search for those social situations that are less demanding.

Behavior	*16. The person is very restless, cannot stay still, or is easily agitated.*
Common Responses	Something is bothering him; he does not have anything to do.
Alzheimer's Interpretation	As the disease progresses, agitation and restlessness commonly accompany the insecurity created by the person's diminishing abilities to cope. De-

nial and rationalization, which previously helped to block out awareness of functional losses, become less successful protective devices as his problems become more pronounced.

Some restlessness may suggest anxiety and underlying fears, though the person cannot always explain these feelings. Too much stimulation can contribute to anxious and agitated behavior. Medication given to control these symptoms should be carefully monitored, as it can sometimes intensify the symptoms it was prescribed to decrease.

Helpful Responses

- Use a calm, reassuring approach that supports his feelings, even when the underlying source is not apparent.

- If he can say what is bothering him, try to eliminate the source of trouble; if he cannot, avoid pressing for explanations.

- Reduce noise and activity levels.

- Ask the physician if the agitation can be decreased with medication or if medication might be creating the undesired effects.

- Involve the person in an activity that helps burn off excess energy.

Behavior
17. The person constantly watches you and follows you around.

Common Responses
She wants too much attention; she is overly dependent; she will not entertain herself; she is suspicious and distrustful of you.

Alzheimer's Interpretation
This problem develops from the fear and insecurity caused by the person's memory impairment; watching or following the caregiver provides greater security. Such behavior also promotes her sense of belonging and alleviates her sense of isolation, which might otherwise intensify anxiety and fear.

Mistrust or suspiciousness may develop because the person is less sure of what is happening. Her interpretations of information and her reasoning capabilities are less reliable. Some persons develop paranoia or more intense suspiciousness as a response to a more threatening world outside themselves.

Helpful Responses

- Understand such behaviors as a search for security.

- Identify and alleviate specific fears that are creating insecurity, for example, the fear that you are leaving the house.

- Orient her as to what is happening and clarify what you are doing.

- Spend time with the person.

- Engage her in constructive activity; ask her to do some supervised things with you.

- Avoid dramatic changes in routine.

Behavior	*18. The person's moods change for no apparent reason. He gets upset and even aggressive if cornered.*
Common Responses	The changes are related to medication, changes in his condition, or something you have done; he is losing his mind and cannot control his emotions.
Alzheimer's Interpretation	Such mood swings are often related to changes in the body and brain as the disease progresses. The mood swings also can be precipitated by thoughts and ideas the person has but is unable or unwilling to express.

The person may also be experiencing a catastrophic reaction, which means that the person is overwhelmed by too much happening too quickly, has become extremely upset by his confusion and loss of control, and cannot respond adequately to the situation.

Helpful Responses

- Consult a physician if significant mood swings occur without cause or are increasing in intensity.

- Remove the person from the upsetting situation slowly and quietly.

- Be realistic in your expectations and avoid pushing.

- Reduce outside stimulants.

- Avoid expressing anger and frustration.

- Avoid reasoning or arguing, but use nonverbal support such as holding hands in a calming fashion.

Behavior	*19. The person refuses to bathe and groom; she says she has already done so.*
Common Responses	She does not care about her personal appearance; she is being stubborn and uncooperative; she is lying.
Alzheimer's Interpretation	Regular bathing and attention to personal hygiene lose their social significance for persons with brain impairment. Social judgment and awareness diminish. Since taking care of per-

sonal hygiene is the most basic sign of independence, however, it becomes threatening to adults to become dependent upon someone's help to bathe and groom themselves.

Bathing can become embarrassing to the brain-impaired person. Being nude, closed in, and helpless in a bathtub or shower creates a sense of vulnerability that may be frightening.

Because the person is accustomed to bathing regularly, it may make perfect sense in her mind to claim she has bathed.

Helpful Responses

- Maintain bathing and grooming at regularly scheduled times.
- Make bathing and grooming comfortable and relaxing experiences; offer, for example, a warm bath and relaxing back massage.
- Be aware of potential fears such as anxiety about falling or water that is too hot.

Behavior	*20. The person fails to recognize familiar persons, places, and things.*
Common Responses	He is getting much worse and is terribly confused.
Alzheimer's Interpretation	Due to a kind of brain impairment known as agnosia, the person is gradually losing his function of recognition. What his eyes see no longer can

be put together into the previously meaningful and understandable picture. Thus people, places, and things he has been around all of his life now truly appear unfamiliar.

**Helpful
Responses**

- Avoid arguing when this occurs, as conflict will increase the person's confusion and fear.
- Agree that things look different and calmly indicate who you are or identify the thing in question.
- Bring specific and recognizable things to the person's attention to help reestablish contact with the past.
- Avoid rushing the person.

Behavior	*21. The person wanders around at night or seems to be looking for something.*
Common Responses	She is confused and does not know what she is doing; she is being inconsiderate.
Alzheimer's Interpretation	Wandering may occur when the person is disoriented in the middle of the night and has forgotten her reason for awakening. The sleeping difficulties may be caused by frightening noises,

hallucinations, or nightmares. When there is a lack of structured daily routine, the difference between night and day is less pronounced.

**Helpful
Responses**

- Reorient the person when she is wandering in the household.
- Reassure the person that she can look for whatever she wants tomorrow, after a good night's sleep.
- Keep a light on in the bathroom.
- Consult a physician if sleeping difficulties persist.
- Increase the person's level of activity during the day.

Behavior	**22. The person refuses to eat, or he eats very little.**
Common Responses	He has a poor appetite; he is too picky about food; he needs to be more active.
Alzheimer's Interpretation	As Alzheimer's progresses, it is common for decreases in appetite to occur. Eating binges and a desire for sweets also occur, but greater concerns are created by the refusal to eat. Often persons

fail to eat because they believe they have already eaten or because they simply forget what they are doing. This is more likely to occur with persons who live alone or in situations where structured daily routine is minimal.

Brain impairment also contributes to difficulties in using eating utensils. Swallowing can be difficult.

Helpful Responses

- Minimize between-meal snacks.
- Maintain as high a level of physical activity as possible.
- Provide regular meals that follow a routine.
- Eat with the person.
- Prepare familiar and favorite foods.
- Be sure food can be easily chewed and swallowed.
- Cut meat as necessary; use utensils that are easy to hold.
- As coordination deteriorates, offer direct assistance.
- Consider using vitamins or food supplements.
- Avoid overemphasizing neat eating habits.
- Give the person more time to eat.

Behavior	**23. The person does not seem to care for you anymore, and she says you do not love or care about her.**

Common Responses	She no longer loves and appreciates you.

Alzheimer's Interpretation	As brain impairment progresses, the person's awareness of the people around her naturally diminishes. She becomes less expressive and makes fewer gestures of appreciation. When she

questions whether you love or care about her, she may be seeking reassurance to counteract her sense that she is losing you due to her diminishing abilities.

Helpful Responses

- Reassure her that you care, without taking offense at her questions.
- Provide as much involvement as possible with other individuals and supporting influences, such as an Alzheimer's Family Support Group.

Behavior	*24. The person's hands and arms shake; he stumbles and is unsteady when he walks.*

Common Responses	He is nervous; he has visual problems; his arthritis is getting worse.

Alzheimer's Interpretation	While nervousness may be responsible for some of the shaking, other causes also should be considered. Side effects of medications prescribed

for severe agitation, delusions, hallucinations, and sleeping problems may be the source. Stiffness also could be caused by these medications.

In other cases, tremors may be directly related to the brain impairment. Rapid jerking movements of the limbs or even the body can occur. These are called myoclonic jerks and should be evaluated by a physician.

Loss of mobility and coordination of large (gross) and small (fine) movements occur with the disease. These coordination problems contribute to difficulties with all motor skills. Weakness, poor balance, and stooped posture make walking difficult; likewise, difficulty in getting up from a chair leads to long periods of sitting. Prompt medical attention should be sought as these conditions escalate.

Some persons with Alzheimer's may exhibit symptoms suggestive of Parkinson's disease. This neurological disorder can coexist with Alzheimer's, but it is difficult to differentiate when Alzheimer's is in its advanced stages.

**Helpful
Responses**

- Check to be sure that poor vision or other impairments do not restrict the person's mobility.

- Change furniture, lighting, throw rugs, and so forth to promote safety at home.

- Provide the person with ample opportunities for exercise to prevent premature weakness and loss of coordination.

- Avoid rushing the person, provide assistance when required, and encourage him to carry out tasks one step at a time.

- Consult a physician when dramatic deterioration in motor skills occurs.

Behavior	*25. The person sits doing nothing for long periods of time.*
Common Responses	She should be doing something worthwhile; she should be more active; she is bored, lazy, or depressed.
Alzheimer's Interpretation	As brain impairment affects memory and intellectual abilities, spontaneous and self-initiated activity diminishes. Apathy and a lack of interest in what is going on develops because the person's

ability to partake in daily life is compromised. Her abilities to plan and carry out purposeful activity are likewise affected by diminished cognitive abilities. Later, she may develop problems with walking and standing. More positively, sitting quietly may be a welcomed relief for her from the increasingly stressful demands of daily life.

**Helpful
Responses**

- Develop daily routines that include enjoyable activities which require minimal concentration.
- Encourage and assist the person's participation in shared activities.
- Walk and exercise with the person to encourage muscle strength and coordination.
- Realize the person may be enjoying the chance to relax and be free of stressful activities.
- Use music and some television to add stimulation to time spent sitting.

Behavior	26. *The person wets or soils himself.*
Common Responses	He is not trying to control his bodily functions and does not care anymore; he wants your attention; he is trying to get back at you for something.
Alzheimer's Interpretation	These problems are not uncommon in more advanced stages of Alzheimer's. The person is less aware of the need to relieve himself and does not associate this need with the bathroom.

Memory problems and perceptual difficulties make it more difficult for the person to find the bathroom. At night, disorientation and confusion make it more difficult to use the bathroom.

**Helpful
Responses**

- Assist the person in maintaining regularly scheduled trips to the bathroom.
- Leave a night light on in the bathroom.
- Consider reducing the intake of liquids in the evening.
- Label the bathroom door and help the person practice finding it.

- Be understanding of bladder and bowel accidents, which are quite embarrassing to the individual.

- Have a doctor examine the person for other underlying medical problems.

Behavior	***27. The person wanders aimlessly.***
Common Responses	She is disoriented and lost; she does not have anything to do.
Alzheimer's Interpretation	Wandering is a problem for people who have brain damage. Because of the potential consequences of wandering, it is a behavior with potentially dangerous outcomes. The person could

fall or become lost in the neighborhood. (We have considered some aspects of wandering in *Behavior 16*, restlessness/agitation and *Behavior 21*, nocturnal confusion.)

Wandering cannot be easily understood if one sees it as aimless. In fact, what appears to be aimless wandering is not an aimless activity at all in many cases. A brain damaged by Alzheimer's disease merely has difficulty determining the purpose or goal of such activity. The impaired person may .not be able to communicate; thus the caregiver cannot arrive at the reasons with questions. In such cases, the caregiver may find that the purpose of the wandering becomes clearer through observation. Often people who are thought to be wandering aimlessly follow the same path repeatedly. This may be more evident in institutional settings. Along that path are sources of positive stimulation (outside views, water, coffee, social contact). Wandering can also be an effort to avoid or escape adversive situations, such as dark or noisy areas and more isolated spots which create a strong sense of insecurity.

Other explanations for what appears to be wandering behavior include the following possibilities.

1. The person is looking for something she has lost.
2. The person does not recognize her surroundings and may be looking for something familiar. (This may be an example of agnosia—failure to recognize familiar persons, things, places— or a reaction to new or changed physical environment.)

3. The person is more confused, restless, or agitated as a reaction to tranquilizers or other medication.

4. The person may be more confused during certain parts of the day, for example, early morning or late evening.

5. The person may be confused as a result of sensory impairment. Because she hears or sees poorly, she cannot comprehend sights and sounds accurately. These types of impairments can also result from brain damage. In this case, the individual cannot process visual and auditory information correctly, and her perceptions are distorted.

6. The person may wander as a response to stress. She may walk away from upsetting situations and then become lost. A catastrophic reaction may precede the wandering behavior. Some persons may have always gotten upset easily by a stressful situation and walked away from it.

Helpful Responses

- First, determine the type of wandering. Is it really aimless, or is the wandering goal-directed?

- Then, determine if the wandering is an attempt to gain something (stimulation, food, drink, security, or physical activity because of restlessness).

- Remember that restlessness and pacing are common during some phases of Alzheimer's disease. Supervise this activity constructively. Walk with the person in a safe and stimulating area. (Too much stimulation can be overwhelming at times.)

- Determine if the wandering behavior is a response to stressful environmental factors. For example, too much noise or demands placed on the person too quickly and forcefully may precipitate behavior that results in wandering and getting lost.

- Determine if the person's apparent wandering is a reaction to fear. Has the individual misinterpreted sights or sounds? Are these delusions or hallucinations? Is she trying to get away from something that frightens her? If so, wandering may be her attempt to seek security and safety. Relate to this need.

- At night, leave some lights on and the door to the bathroom open, so the person does not get lost on the way to the bathroom.

- If you believe the wandering is created by medications, consult your physician for a medications review.

- Place locks on outside doors that cannot be undone by the organically impaired person but which you can open easily.

- Have the person wear a MedAlert-type bracelet which says "memory impaired." A name, phone number, and address on this or some other items will also be helpful.

- If wandering continues to be difficult to manage, consult a physician or mental health professional.

Wandering is a major source of stress to most caregivers. Understandably they worry about it because of its potential harmful outcomes. Caregivers should take action to deal with this problem, or it will create more stress and heighten the need for supervision considerably. If the memory-impaired person does wander away from home, notify the police department immediately. Having pictures of the person along with an accurate description of such characteristics as hair color, height, weight, and other identifiers will increase the chances of the person's being found quickly. Be sure to tell the police that the person is memory impaired, confused, and so forth. You may offer suggestions on how the person may best be approached. If you know, tell police about the status of the person when she left. Was the person upset and angry? It may be better for the caregiver to remain home and have family or friends assist with the search so that someone is at the home should the patient return there.

When the person returns home, it will be better to relate positively to the return. Your anger or scolding will only make matters worse. The person will probably be frightened anyway.

12

GETTING HELP

Few people would argue that more resources need to be developed to assist persons with Alzheimer's disease and family caregivers. Family caregivers—spouses, children, siblings, or other relatives—provide most of the care received by relatives over long periods of time. Often, these individuals make personal sacrifices to take care of their loved ones. They may give up jobs, leisure activities, other family roles, social roles, or relationships. Many gradually let go of activities and roles that had been meaningful for much of a lifetime: church, social clubs, friends, and hobbies.

Getting appropriate help can be a way of softening the impact of caregiving, and lightening the burdens of caring. Sometimes caregivers are at a disadvantage. It is not always clear what kind of help they need, or what help is available. Some help is designed for caregivers; some is designed for their loved ones. They may feel that some problems must be endured; nothing helps. The importance of getting help is not a matter of how much or how often caregivers seek it. The "importance" of getting help lies in how reliable and adequate one perceives that help to be.

Help must be available　　Family members, friends, and professionals who have been involved often urge family caregivers to get help. A prerequisite for getting help would appear to be having someone or something available "when" help is needed. "Help" in this sense might be a product—identification bracelets, alarms on doors, special locks, and medications. A caregiver might seek help in the form of a service—respite, adult day care, and home health care. If respite services were available for a caregiver who is physically and emotionally overwhelmed, then that caregiver could call and set up a respite service. He or she could then benefit from much needed rest and relaxation, knowing their loved one was receiving proper care. If needed products or services are available, all one must do is find them, call about them, and purchase or meet eligibility requirements for them. Getting help "seems" to be a simple matter, but that is far from the case.

Getting Help: The Process of Change

Something is wrong with this simple formula for getting help. Many caregivers seem to resist the very idea of getting help. Some seem to hear concerned people saying the caregiver needs help because they cannot handle the job. Other caregivers try to get help but find there are just too many obstacles to overcome: help might cost too much, the service is too troublesome to arrange, they don't have time to get the help, or persons with Alzheimer's will not cooperate. Perhaps it is better to leave things just as they are. Maybe getting help isn't so simple after all.

Other factors involved If help is available and the caregiver wants help, then they should be able to get help with little trouble. However, this approach did not work in the case of Ginger Haught. Other factors interfered.

Ginger is 62 years old; she is married and has a son. Her family lives about 15 miles outside of Waco, Texas. Her mother, Clara, who lives in the same rural area, has exhibited symptoms commonly associated with Alzheimer's disease for the past four years. Some of the symptoms have become more pronounced. Her memory is worse; she refuses to bathe.

Ginger, her son, and a supportive sister have tried to get Clara to see her family doctor on many occasions. To Clara it was outrageous that her family would insist she see a doctor. There was nothing wrong with her. Just a waste of time and money—two things Clara had resisted wasting since birth. Ginger and the rest of the family knew that Mom would continue to have the last word on this matter. If they pressured her, she would become more aggravated and less cooperative with other things. Her mother forgot so many important things—eating and turning the gas heater off—but never seemed to forget the things that made her angry.

How can you help someone who doesn't want it, but clearly needs it? Ginger recalled the hurt that had always resulted from previous disagreements with her mother. This time the situation was different. Her mother wasn't doing well. Still, she felt responsible for her mother's condition. Getting help was so frustrating. She felt guilty because she couldn't find a good solution to her dilemma, or one acceptable to her mother. What should she do? Who helps you with guilt and frustration?

Beliefs for change

This dilemma is all too familiar to many family caregivers. Alzheimer's is not like other diseases. It changes the degree of a loved one's legitimate participation in decision making. Reasoning with your family member doesn't seem to work anymore. "White lies" or other creative strategies might be substituted, and then it might be possible for a loved one to be seen for a professional evaluation. Although these approaches can be effective, caregivers using them feel like they are deceiving or betraying loved ones. They feel guilty and anticipate that greater difficulties in providing care might result. Doing something against a loved one's will represents a breach in trust. It seems to go against the beliefs on which relationships are built.

When caregivers seek help, appropriate resources to help them must be both available and accessible. Ginger believed her mother needed to see a doctor. The doctor was probably available, but if her mother agreed to see him, he would need to see her before she changed her mind again. Being successful in getting help means using momentum to your advantage. Being accessible meant that if she called to talk with him, she couldn't wait four hours, or talk to three other people first. If Ginger succeeded in getting her mother to the doctor's office, he would need to see her immediately. She might change her mind in the waiting room. This could cause an argument and make a "scene" in front of everyone. The doctor might even refuse to see Clara.

Old needs persist

Ginger was quite aware she had never gotten the approval she needed from her mother. Clara had always been critical of Ginger and her husband. It had always been difficult for them to handle any type of conflict constructively. Ginger found the accusations and anger that resulted from these conflicts very painful. In her own mind, she believed there was a catastrophe ahead—even if she were able to get her mother to the doctor. Sometimes it seems so many things must work "just right" when you are trying to help loved ones. If they don't, nothing gets done.

New basis for needs

Anticipate and plan for difficulties that can be reasonably expected. The fact these difficulties occur doesn't mean we must react to them in habitual ways. For example, Ginger does not have to argue with her mother as she did in the past. Arguing with a person with Alzheimer's disease makes situations worse. Ginger must also have the opportunity to see that her mother's behavior may no longer be influenced by problems in their relationship. Other caregivers may, like Ginger, be influenced by old beliefs about behavior and why things happen. These beliefs may be the source of self-defeating thoughts. Emotional reactions resulting from these beliefs obscure the options that remain. The personalities of loved ones influenced how they handled problems before. Now the effects of brain impairment also influences their responses to problems, and your attempts to solve them.

Role in helping changes

Changing beliefs about loved ones' capabilities to make good choices is difficult. It is confusing to separate what is the willful expression of personality from the more unintentional behavior resulting from brain damage. Our beliefs about responsible adults getting help are based on ideas that are associated with normal functioning and intention. But Ginger realizes her mother's behavior isn't responsible. She is also aware of the history of her mother's behavior, especially as it relates to her. If the mental anguish of not helping becomes more intense than the fears of what will happen if she does something, then Ginger will eventually act.

Dramatic change in roles

To family members assuming a helping role, it is quite a leap from knowing loved ones will take care of problems themselves to making decisions on their behalf. It may be necessary for Ginger to take a greater leap since long-standing problems exist in the relationship she has had with her mother. Her involvement seems to depend upon her mother giving her approval for Ginger to act on her behalf. Getting help would be easier if this were true. However, Ginger, and other caregivers in this dilemma, need to modify this expectation and seek permission from other sources. Family support may be sufficient, yet professional help may be necessary if family members cannot agree on what must be done, and the primary caregiver is uncomfortable acting alone.

Another view helps   The help from the doctor might not have been the place to start. Ginger did not understand that other means of getting her mother to the doctor—inappropriate as they were before—might be acceptable in the present situation. Maybe there were services or other people who could help her resolve her conflict. Ginger finally attended an Alzheimer's family support group. There she learned the problem that had seemed so unique was really quite common. The encouragement she received was invaluable at a demoralizing point in getting help for her mother. Professional consultants to the group reinforced the information she had received from other individuals in the group.

Decision to act   It would be difficult, but now she knew what she must do. She knew other caregivers had had similar difficulties. If things didn't go smoothly, that was to be expected. If her mother was upset with her, she wouldn't allow that to bother her so much. Ginger's son could help. Now she had a group of people who understood what must be done, and who listened to her. She was becoming a caregiver. Doubt and frustration might be common experiences. She will feel hurt and anger; guilt may always be in the back of her mind. But "she has choices" about what she does and how she feels. Her beliefs about getting help extend beyond the help she will need specifically for her mother. She has given herself permission to seek help for herself. And that is quite appropriate for what lies ahead. Her mother will benefit.

Realistic helpers   It is essential that caregivers receive help from people who have a realistic view of how to deal with what is happening. Caregivers can be creative in adapting to their own situations. They can be resourceful in meeting the demands they face without the assistance of outside help, although outside help may be needed to get them started and support them along the way. Getting help should result in support of family caregiving, but not at the expense of family involvement. Providers of this help must perceive the needs of the "whole picture" of care. This view includes both victims, not only the "patient" or the "caregiver." It must also consider other factors that prevail on the decision to get help.

Address the old problems

Before seeking help for problems moré clearly associated with Alzheimer's disease, caregivers may need to address other problems that represent barriers to getting help. This may be the more difficult initial step in caregiving. It will involve changing the ways one has related to a family member before the symptoms of Alzheimer's appeared. It was the most difficult step for Ginger to take. Getting diagnostic evaluations are also difficult for some of the same reasons she experienced: the relative doesn't want to go and doesn't see any reason for an evaluation since there are really no problems. The fact the loved one is afraid may not occur to you.

Decision-making stress

If you become responsible for a loved one who has always made the decisions in your family, it may be as difficult to "make" the decisions as it is to carry them out. Wives who had assumed a more submissive role in the relationship with their husbands, and who had been dependent upon their husbands to make decisions for them, can be quite uncomfortable making big decisions when they begin to deal with the responsibilities of caregiving. Caregivers who are spouses begin to make decisions with less, or less dependable input from marital partners. Responses to needs in the present may be based on attitudes and preferences carried over from the past that are incongruent with current problems and needs.

Influence of family

Pre-existing marital relationships influence caregiving and help-seeking. So do other family interactions. Relations with other family members may be strained when everyone does not view the situation and what is needed in the same way. Children who become active caregivers may be forced to confront problems in the relationships with their parents before getting help. This is quite evident in the previous example. Siblings may be faced with the challenge of communicating when they have differences—old, new, or reactivated—that stand in the way of responding to the needs of the relative with Alzheimer's disease.

Families are unique. Some family characteristics may make it more difficult for that family to deal with Alzheimer's disease. Some families do seem to have more problems meeting the demands of caregiving than others. The primary caregiver in a disengaged family can probably expect less support in seeking outside help. He or she can also expect less support from within the family. The caregiver in an enmeshed family may be more reluctant to seek outside help since everyone in the family is so involved in influencing what should happen. Family interactions may create barriers to getting help. The fact that some families handle situations differently does not mean there is one right way for care to be provided. What works in one family may create a disaster in another.

Addressing Emotional Needs

Alzheimer's differs from other diseases. Most of the symptoms suggest a psychiatric or neurological disorder, yet these symptoms could be attributed to other causes before they become more pronounced or cause other persistent problems in daily living. Problems with memory or small changes in personality are not addressed in the same way as severe headaches or loss of movement and undeniable confusion. Since the earlier behavioral symptoms may vary considerably in intensity and duration, they can be attributed to stress or problems in a relationship. It is common for relatives to look back after the tentative diagnosis of Alzheimer's disease is given and recall much earlier suspicions that something was wrong. They are able to understand why the behaviors or emotional episodes in the past might have occurred. These questionable events fall into place and make sense once relatives have a new perspective from which to interpret them.

Family members may feel guilty they did not act sooner to find out why their loved ones were acting out of character. Delaying the evaluation didn't cause the disease. As in Ginger's example, many family members realized something was wrong. They did not have any idea of how to proceed, particularly since it is common for persons who are developing Alzheimer's disease to deny or be unaware of the problems others observe. That means family members must contradict their loved one's perception of the problem. Even though they may be aware of the difficulties they are alleged to have, fear of what might be wrong is too difficult to confront. Some of these individuals may be confused about what might be happening. More than one individual given a diagnosis of Alzheimer's disease has been relieved by this news. They were much more afraid of having a psychiatric disorder.

Ambiguous losses Alzheimer's disease leads to a psychological death long before relatives recognize aspects of deterioration that imminently suggest a physical death. This ambiguity makes grieving more difficult and postpones its finality. It also makes it more difficult for caregivers to know when to get help, or what kind of help to seek. It is estimated that more than 30 percent of persons with Alzheimer's disease suffer from clinical depression. A larger percentage have features of clinical depression.

If depression is present, the victim of the illness may benefit from treatment. Excess disabilities associated with the effects of the depressive illness can be minimized. This can reduce some demands on the caregiver. For the Alzheimer's victim, this treatment may assist with improved mood, coping, and less difficulty in performing activities of daily living. Smaller improvements in cognitive abilities might occur. In addition to treatment based primarily on the administration of antidepressant medications, more effective applications of cognitive/behavioral therapy (Teri and Gallagher-Thompson 1991; Gallagher et al. 1989) are being developed for victims and their families.

Caring for an individual with Alzheimer's disease is likely to be a physically, emotionally, and spiritually challenging endeavor. The significance of the "emotional burden" alone cannot be minimized. Caregiving can lead to such emotional responses as denial, anger, guilt, self-pity, and depression (Oliver and Bock 1985). Estimates of the percentage of caregivers experiencing depression vary, yet it is apparent that as many as 45 percent do experience depression (Gallagher et al. 1989).

Coping differs   Women seem to experience higher rates than men (Pruchno and Resch 1989), but this difference may be less than expected (Gallagher et al. 1989). Differences in coping styles may account for women being more vulnerable than men to the stresses of caregiving. Men may use more outside help for things like housekeeping and personal care of their wives. Wives may be more emotionally involved in the relationship. The loss of the relationship may prove more difficult than daily caregiving.

Treat both   Inconsistencies in research prevent generaliza-
depressions   tions about why a caregiver wife might have a higher risk than a husband caring for his wife. There may be too many individual factors involved. The nature of depression, and the serious impact it can have on the lives of persons with Alzheimer's and their caregivers cannot be ignored. When caregivers actively seek help for the burdens and stresses that affect their lives, they may be suffering from depression half of the time (Gallagher, Rose et al. 1989). Both the family member needing care and his or her caregiver may develop depression. Help should be sought since both could benefit from treatment. Caregiving will be more manageable.

Dynamics of Caregiving

Caregiving is not a static experience. It is as dynamic as the disease process it addresses. One study of this dynamic process found that caregivers experienced more symptoms suggesting mental health problems and depression near the time of a nursing home placement and the six-month period following the placement (Lichtenberg and Barth 1989). Nursing home placement is one of several psychosocial events that occur during the caregiving process that are likely to be associated with greater shock, stress, and grief. It does not make the experience of caring any easier.

Health problems of caregivers or other family members add to the stress and burden of caring for a loved one. These situations may represent transitional points in caregiving when families will benefit from outside help. Seeking help need not be a constant activity, but caregivers must recognize changing needs that require a response.

More dramatic and persistent behavioral changes might be related to the normal progression of the disease. Such changes can be associated with environmental conditions or changes in the caregiver's relationship with a loved one. They may also indicate underlying medical problems or more severe psychiatric problems. Incontinence may be directly related to the disease progression. It might indicate a medical problem. For example, urinary tract, bladder, or yeast infections are examples of less serious medical problems that may be heralded by more intense behavioral or psychiatric manifestations.

Reduce your concerns

Medications may be helpful, but side effects can masquerade as more dramatic deterioration. Accessible physicians will be able to address medical concerns. Excess disability and unnecessary discomfort or pain can be minimized. Stress related to the concerns of the caregivers can be reduced. Timely consultation with professionals also allows caregivers to have their own needs addressed.

Psychiatric changes

Neurological and more severe psychiatric symptoms that appear for the first time may be both frightening and difficult for caregivers to manage. The development of delusions may catch some caregivers off guard. Some delusions are difficult to accept or understand. Accusations of caregivers having affairs are not uncommon. The person with dementia will act as though this were really happening, which creates behavior management problems. Caregivers may be able to handle some psychiatric problems. Others may disrupt their ability to function as much as they disturb loved ones.

Anxious and agitated behavior may result from delusional ideas that relatives develop. Activities of daily living will be more troublesome to complete. Sleeping problems often develop when delusional ideas persist. Caregivers will have their sleep disturbed. Professionals may be able to help caregivers understand the fears that are associated with delusions and some hallucinations. They sometimes provide valuable clues about the internal emotional experiences of loved ones. If psychiatric symptoms are bothersome to either caregivers or their loved ones, and are fairly persistent, caregivers need to consider getting help from medical or mental health professionals.

Grief's Impact on Getting Help

Grief affects the entire family in Alzheimer's caregiving. The victim experiences grief, at least until the ability to reason, think, and remember is gone. Some of the behavioral and emotional reactions caregivers find difficult to manage or respond to sensitively may be expressions of a "mourning of the self" in their loved ones. Unfortunately, this grieving process is seldom completed before it is halted by greater brain-related impairment.

Caregivers don't fare much better because their own process of grieving is constantly suspended by new demands. The physical death is slow and extremely unpredictable. The scriptural image of the "valley of the shadow of death" aptly captures the presence of both the psychological and physical deaths that face caregivers. Even when their own need to grieve is suspended by the demands of the moment, the shadow of death stretches over their lives and the lives of those they love. And yet the needs of sustaining a relationship are met in caregiving activities that bond them closer to loved ones. Caregivers can become so involved in the lives of loved ones that they have difficulty separating their own emotions, identities, and individual sense of well-being from loved ones (Rose and DelMaestro 1990).

Fear of separation

Caregivers can find help for many of the problems they encounter during caregiving. There is no help that prevents their losses, only help for getting over them. It is extremely threatening to participate in the kind of separation caused by Alzheimer's disease. Wives, for instance, may sense they are "letting go" when they must make decisions for a husband who is no longer psychologically present to guide and support them (Gwyther 1990). Asking for help, especially when they have never had to ask for it outside the marriage before, is an acknowledgment of a loss that will erode the sense of "we-ness" that had been validated by the relationship of marriage.

All healthy adult relationships have a certain degree of the kind of involvement that is associated with this "oneness." The idea of marriage is based on beliefs that two people become one. Healthy dependencies can exist in this relationship, particularly when the individuals involved maintain boundaries that support independent and individual areas of existence. The individual who becomes a caregiver may be challenged by the competing needs to remain separate and become more involved. They must assume responsibility for everything about a loved one's existence. The familiar give-and-take is progressively out of balance. A relationship, a partner, is being lost. Letting go of the sharing of tasks may be the beginning of a prolonged period of anticipatory grief and bereavement. Loved ones who become less of themselves must have more of you.

This process of the caregiver merging with a loved one seems to be a common human response to an anticipated loss. The long "good-bye" so often associated with the Alzheimer's experience is not merely referring to how long it takes for a shadow to embody the one you love. It must also refer to your attachment, and the pain that lingers in the letting go. This bond, which is so like the symbiosis of a mother with her child, is protected, sometimes fiercely so. It can become a formidable barrier to caregivers reaching out for help and concerned friends, family members, and professionals getting in to help (Rose and DelMaestro 1990; Gwyther 1990; Lewin and Lundervold 1990).

Finding a balance, as a part of the process of letting go, must be appreciated by the caregivers and the professional helpers who are obstructed. This symbiosis becomes a relationship with well-guarded boundaries. We can all recall stories that describe the self-sacrificing nature of this relationship in the animal world. Those that tell of the mother being destroyed to protect her young are touching. Even in the world of people, stories of mothers dying to protect their children, reveal our feelings about this "special" relationship.

A return to a symbiotic relationship with a spouse or parent, when their lives are threatened by Alzheimer's disease, doesn't continue to elicit these feelings once the bonding becomes destructive. It has potential for creating a "loss of self" in the caregiver. In these cases, the symbiotic relationship becomes a vessel of bondage from which one cannot or does not seek escape. To break it may seem like one is declaring the end to any relationship at all.

Refuge for finishing and healing	Since symbiosis reflects one's need to hold loved ones closer and keep them longer, it is a normal thing to do. In this sense, the "vessel of bondage" serves as a temporary, but necessary refuge until the meaning of the disease and its impact on

one's life can be absorbed. Then one leaves it more willingly. The reluctance to leave and be separate might be viewed as the caregiver's wish to "responsibly finish" their relationship (Gwyther 1990).

This has its parallel in the mother-child symbiosis. Mothers find it extremely difficult to release their children from the protective bond that connects them. Children must be allowed to separate and face the world. If they are constrained by the attachment with the mother, they cannot grow and develop normally. They would be unable to become secure, reasonably independent individuals in adulthood. Some mothers hold on longer to be certain their relationship is reasonably finished. Others hold on indefinitely because they cannot emotionally tolerate the separation from their "child." The child may be reluctant to leave if he perceives his mother's existence depends solely on him.

Conflicts   In a sense, caregivers experience the need of the
letting go   mother to "hold on." In another way, caregivers
                  resemble the child who needs to separate, but
fears the separation will endanger the loved one who has become vulnerable. In this context, separation is synonymous with abandonment. Who would dare abandon a child? Social injunctions against this are very strong. Caregivers who view loved ones as children are more likely to suffer the bondage of symbiosis. They may perceive outside help as an intrusion.

Letting Go

The conflicts family caregivers experience around becoming separate from relatives who are very slowly dying may account for their reluctance to use available help. It may affect their decision to get help very early, and persist when letting go seems impossible. Outside help poses a threat to the relationship one is attempting to preserve. This might be expected to have grater influence on older spouses who become caregivers (Gwyther 1990). Their relationships that have existed longer. The future without a life-long partner may be more frightening to comprehend.

A number of caregiver beliefs reflect their difficulties viewing themselves as separate individuals. One example is their inability to accept the intellectual impairment of loved ones as "real" (Rose and DelMaestro 1990). The idea that loved ones are not like they used to be is unacceptable. It threatens the symbiotic identify found in the relationship with the loved one who is impaired. To suggest that one is impaired implies "we" are not like we used to be.

This belief is reinforced by another: the well-being of the caregiver and "patient" are rigidly interdependent. What happens to one happens to the other. If the impaired family member is sad and unhappy, and the caregiver is asked about her own feelings, she might say "He's not doing well," or, "We've been down lately." The caregiver cannot separate her feelings or herself from the loved one who isn't the same. For these reasons, caregivers are unwilling to allow others to help them. After a nursing home placement, they continue to spend most of their time with loved ones. When they receive in-home respite, they remain at home to be certain "they" are alright.

Difficulties resolving the conflict to become a separate individual again occur in healthy families and marriages. They may be more difficult to address in relationships where issues of independence and dependence, being separate and overly involved, persist. Any caregiver will find it very hard to maintain any emotional distance from a loved one once the consequences of Alzheimer's disease are considered. Some will reach a point in which emotional withdrawal is desired. Emotional "distancing" is a type of self-protection for the caregiver. The supportive presence of the caregiver is important to their loved one. Withdrawal must be gradual, or it will be detrimental to the person experiencing the disease. They will sense emotional ties are being severed. Professional help may contribute to the resolution of these conflicts at a time when that resolution is especially important.

Death's reality a real fear Intellectual and psychological losses pose a serious threat to the "symbiotic" bond. Threats of physical death begin to be encountered as "real" in the later stages of the disease. Caregivers who had fears they were abandoning loved ones as psychological death became apparent, may be troubled by these anxieties again when their physical "wasting away" becomes apparent. Now Alzheimer's has the look of a legitimate medical disease. Caregivers who might have been achieving a healthier degree of separation may find themselves drawn back to loved ones. A new "separation" crisis develops.

"Lazarus syndrome"   Assuming other medical conditions are not life-threatening, Alzheimer's disease itself leads to death. Dying can be very slow, and marked by periods of apparent remission or slight improvements. In the advanced stages of the disease, caregivers will see behavioral and physical changes that suggest the ordeal will end soon. They prepare for this final separation, and loved ones keep living. This phenomena, call the "Lazarus syndrome" (Rando 1984), is common in chronic and progressive diseases such as Alzheimer's disease. Caregivers may feel angry or ambivalent. After several episodes during which loved ones hold onto life, they may feel guilty because they wish the separation to be complete.

Grief and the future   Caregivers have provided for the needs of loved ones. They have lived with uncertainty, and responded the best they could. They were aware that the death of their loved one was the one thing that was certain. Its finality may not be so certain. The future has been difficult to consider, yet the time comes for caregivers to consider their future. This is also the time when the grieving that has been suspended can continue, and be completed.

The tasks of grief   For survivors, one of the goals of grieving is to establish a new identity separate from the deceased. Developing a new identity requires emancipation from the bondage of the deceased (Rando 1984). In Alzheimer's disease, overly attached caregivers need to find ways to begin this process earlier. Bondage to a loved one who had been psychologically absent, but physically present, remains after physical death. The process of grief is a process of healing. To heal, one must accept the reality of the loss and work through the associated pain. This also involves adjusting to a world from which the deceased is missing. Finally, the survivor will need to emotionally relocate the deceased and move on with life (Worden 1991). In this sense, the idea of getting help is getting yourself back again.

Becoming Yourself Again

Getting help is not always a process with clear direction toward tangible goals. Getting help involves one's perception of the problem, and a determination of how it can best be addressed. Many of the challenges of Alzheimer's care don't result from problems and needs that can be so easily identified or solved. Getting help may be another way to address this ambiguity. Then it becomes a process that leads toward finding meaning in one's own suffering, and finding some better way to understand the loss of a relationship to a disease that has neither cure nor known cause. Getting help is one way to be sure you have done all that can be done, and knowing you have done it as well as anyone in your situation.

Finally, the process of getting help may encourage you to become a unique individual again as you reconstruct a separate future. Caregivers who are grieving will experience a broad range of physical, emotional, and behavioral changes in themselves. Grief will also manifest itself in their thoughts. If they are unfamiliar with grief, some caregivers will fear they are losing their minds. A few will even fear they are developing Alzheimer's disease. Their experiences during caregiving do not necessarily prepare them for dealing with both the loss of a loved one and what seems to be a loss of themselves.

They need not fear grief if they permit it to be a process of healing. This involves successful completion of grief through painful, but meaningful, work. It is an active process that one becomes involved in instead of resisting. Individual growth and development can occur. Both are enriched by what you have experienced and the persons who have been involved in that experience. Some of these persons can help you move on into life again. The Alzheimer's experience will finally be finished when your grief is over. You are on your own, again. This is different from the time you left the security of a mother's love. You have learned a great deal since that separation. Now you must become yourself again with yesterday's memories. The future beckons you.

13

EXPLORING COMMUNITY RESOURCES

Some communities have better resources than others. Since the early 1980s, Alzheimer's disease has received considerable public attention. The media has given particular emphasis to the impact this illness has on both its victims and their families. Nonetheless, most communities do not have services and care facilities developed specifically for the long-term needs of Alzheimer's patients. Nor do they provide support services for the family; for example, not all communities have sufficient day and respite programs which address the needs of both patient and caregiver. However, most communities do have agencies that provide for the various long-term care needs of the elderly, and these agencies often provide support and service to Alzheimer's patients and caregivers.

Drawing upon community resources reduces strain on the caregiver. Throughout this book, the importance of calling upon community resources has been stressed. In this chapter, the creative and appropriate use of these resources will be discussed in more detail. Such resources can allow the family to care for the Alzheimer's victim at home without a severely restrictive quality of life. The caregiver has been described as the hidden victim of this illness, and his needs cannot be ignored. But the physical and mental strain placed on the caregiver can be significantly reduced if both family and community resources are sufficiently utilized.

Families need to plan ahead and to explore community resources before the need becomes critical. Family members may feel at first that they prefer to manage alone. But community resources become more important as the primary caregiver grows more isolated and fatigued. Interest in exploring other resources naturally develops as the caregiver begins to wonder how much longer he can continue in the caregiver role. A need for outside help will also surface as the patient's deterioration produces greater difficulties in management and self-care. It is therefore advisable that families explore the resources available in their communities in the early stages of the disease, so they are prepared when the eventual need for more help arises. Families equipped with facts about what lies ahead find it easier to anticipate and plan for the future.

Finding out about helpful services The first step in utilizing community resources is to identify what resources exist. The following are some good places to begin when searching for the resources in your community.

- *Health Professionals.* Family physicians, psychiatrists, mental health professionals, social workers, and others already involved with the Alzheimer's patient are a natural starting point. Ask them for referrals and resource suggestions to address the needs and problems at hand.

- *Community Mental Health Centers.* Mental health centers that have services for the elderly or offer more specialized Alzheimer's care can be a valuable information resource. These agencies can work with the person who has Alzheimer's and his family or spouse. After determining the types of resources needed, the agency can link families with the services that exist in the community.

- *Area Agencies on Aging.* These agencies are involved in developing community resources supportive of the needs of the aging population. Persons with Alzheimer's represent a special part of this population, and area agencies on aging are likely to be knowledgeable about local resources that will support Alzheimer's care.

- *Medical Information and Referral Programs.* These programs exist to aid persons seeking information about and help with medical conditions of all kinds. They may be attached to a governmental agency, a care facility, or a program for the elderly. To locate such a program in your community, contact a medical facility or the Agency on Aging.

- *Alzheimer's Resource and Information Centers.* More recently, some communities have developed programs that specifically address the resource and informational needs of the Alzheimer's patient and family. Such programs may survey the individuals' needs and help caregivers manage their situations. They also may refer the family to other community social-service or mental-health programs developed for the aged or persons with Alzheimer's.

- *Alzheimer's Family Support Groups.* These groups provide important information about more formal local resources that support the care of the Alzheimer's patient. Such groups also may provide information about individuals who can be hired to stay with the person in the home and help with personal care and supervision.

Developing goals for caregiving   Once the family knows the full range of resources available, members can choose the ones most helpful in their situation. In determining how to use resources, the family may wish to reflect on the goals of caregiving. Often, the overall goal of caregiving is to keep the relative in the familiar surroundings of his home. However, refining this goal can provide the caregiver with more definite guidelines for selecting community resources. He should draw upon those that can help him to:

1. *Maintain the patient's social and self-care abilities at the highest possible level.* Premature dependencies place an excessive strain on the family caregiver. To maintain the person's abilities, an appropriate degree of social activity and stimulation is needed, which the family cannot always provide.

2. *Support the patient's adjustment to the gradual losses and limitations associated with the illness.* Persons with Alzheimer's can benefit from supportive counseling, particularly in the

disease's earlier stages, and they can appreciate emotional support for their adjustment throughout. Opportunities for the patient to continue in familiar activities with some degree of success are needed. These successes help support the patient's self-esteem and offset other losses that occur.

3. *Support the family's adjustment to the degenerative process of the disease and the stresses of care.* Family members may need supportive counseling to come to grips with the illness and to learn to work supportively with one another. The ongoing activity of caregiving must be supported to avoid the emotional and physical breakdown associated with stress.

4. *Maintain the safest and most supportive environment.* Basic needs must be provided for, and the person must be safe from danger, neglect, abuse, or exploitation. These concerns particularly apply to persons who live alone.

5. *Provide relief from the constant responsibility of caregiving.* Relief from constant supervision of the person, for example, may be possible when a nurse aide assists a few hours a day with personal care and housekeeping. Caregivers can use outside resources to care for their relative, providing opportunities to take care of their own needs.

Guidelines for using resources

Community resources are meant to support, not replace family involvement. In relying on community services, family members should follow these guidelines.

- Ask questions to clarify your understanding of the situation.
- Express your own needs and concerns.
- Use contact with one community resource as an opportunity to learn about other resources that might be helpful.
- Seek information provided from community resources and professionals when making difficult decisions.

Some community resources that are helpful in caring for Alzheimer's are discussed in the following section. The "Service/Resource" worksheet has been included in the appendix for caregivers to use in comparing and selecting resources.

Community Resources for Alzheimer's Care

1. *Alzheimer's Family Support Groups.* These groups provide caregivers with support in coping with the illness and in dealing with problems experienced in caregiving. Self-support groups also can be a source of information about the disease and community resources. Participants experience similar problems and assist each other in making decisions about care. The emotional adjustment of the family to the illness is promoted by such groups.

2. *Respite Care.* This type of service provides family members with occasional relief from the pressures of continuous caregiving. Such relief can prevent premature institutionalization of the patient as a result of the caregiver's physical and emotional stress. Formal respite programs offer services ranging from several hours' to several weeks' relief.

Respite care also occurs when families hire persons to relieve them from duties in the home. Some families are able to take turns caregiving. In other situations, respite comes as a secondary benefit of medical or psychiatric hospitalizations.

3. *Shared Respite Care.* A number of families with Alzheimer's victims may join together to provide caregiving on a rotating basis. Typically, several family members watch over a group of patients to allow others to have some free time. Benefits are experienced as the Alzheimer's patient and spouse participate with other patients and their families in an activity setting outside the household. By caring for their loved one in company with others, caregivers find that social isolation is reduced. The burden of providing activities becomes an opportunity that is shared by participants.

4. *Adult Day Care.* Some day programs are designed specifically for persons with Alzheimer's. Others provide structured activities to a more heterogeneous group of impaired older persons or other age groups. Day care provides exercise, activities, recreation, support of daily living skills, counseling, and monitoring of the participant's general health. Such programs can help the person with Alzheimer's maintain some abilities that would otherwise deteriorate more quickly. Some provide more specialized social work, nursing, or physical and occupational therapy services. By utilizing adult day care, family members can remain employed, do errands, rest, and be involved in other important areas of their lives.

5. *Home Health Care.* Home health programs usually can provide nursing and personal care services to patients in their homes. For persons with Alzheimer's disease, nursing care is usually not needed until the later stages of the illness, unless other coexisting medical problems exist. But supervision and personal care are very important needs of the Alzheimer's patient. Many home health programs have nurse aids, homemakers, or care providers that can assist with these needs. Self-employed persons also can be hired to provide supervision and assist with the person's personal care needs. Persons with Alzheimer's will definitely need this type of care when they live alone and have no family who live nearby. Home health personnel can help with a broad array of supervisory and direct care needs such as meals and shopping, medications, cleaning and washing, transportation, appraisal of the person's condition, and companionship.

6. *Legal Services.*   Often family members must consider questions such as the person's ability to handle finances and make decisions for himself. Protection of the person and property must be considered, but not at the expense of his other rights and privileges. Alzheimer's disease does not automatically make a person incompetent. When some form of legal guardianship is being considered, the opinion of the treating physician, a psychiatrist, or other mental health professional should be solicited prior to legal consultation.

7. *Community Mental Health Centers.*   Some community mental health centers have specialized geriatric programs that can be very helpful in the management of the Alzheimer's client and supportive of the family caregiver. These programs can provide a wide range of services, including comprehensive assessment, psychiatric evaluations, individual, group, and family counseling. Additionally, case-management services identify other community resources that can help with home maintenance. Referrals can be made and service linkages developed.

Some persons with Alzheimer's disease may present serious behavior management problems. Even when such problems are not apparent, however, the caregiver may find mental health centers helpful in planning care.

Mental health intervention may help in cases of an especially lengthy period of caregiving, a patient with difficult personality traits, a difficult living environment, or other large-scale problems.

Among the specific behaviors that indicate a need for immediate attention are the following:

- Hallucinations and delusions that contribute to sleeping disturbances, agitated and combative behavior, or disruptive interactions with neighbors and community.
- Severe confusion and disorientation.
- Physically threatening behavior.
- Harmful resistance to necessary care and management.
- Potentially dangerous activities such as wandering, driving, and so forth that the family cannot stop.
- Depressive symptoms early in the course of the illness.
- Anxiety, agitation, or denial so extreme that they make care management difficult.

Needs that can be addressed by a mental health center's case-management services include:

- Severe lack of family support.
- High level of caregiver stress.
- An inadequate caregiving situation, such as that of a person who lives alone.

8. *Psychiatric Hospitals.*   Private psychiatric hospitals offer assessment and behavior stabilization. They may be the best resort in cases of unmanageable behavior. The hospital staff can often assist the family with care planning and management.

Considerations for Nursing Home Care

Reevaluating appropriateness of in-home care
Families can use other resources to maintain the loved one in the home. However, conditions may develop that require family members to reexamine the appropriateness of in-home care. Usually these conditions are beyond one's control. Professionals can assist families in deciding whether to

place the person with Alzheimer's disease in a nursing home. The following questions should be considered.

1. Can the total needs of the loved one be adequately provided for on a 24-hour basis in the home?

2. Has the health status of the individual changed so that more nursing care and medical monitoring are necessary?

3. Is the stamina of the caregiver severely taxed by the care situation in the home?

4. If the person lives alone, is there adequate supervision and assistance available to provide for his needs on an ongoing basis?

5. Is it realistic to expect the family to deliver or purchase the services the relative now needs in the home?

6. Are the financial resources of the spouse becoming severely threatened?

7. Do health concerns for the caregiver begin to rival those for the Alzheimer's patient?

8. Has the caregiver's isolation become severe?

9. Is the in-home care contributing to the emotional/physical breakdown of the caregiver/spouse?

10. Is the nursing home placement as unacceptable as it first seemed?

11. Will the quality of contact with the Alzheimer's victim improve by placement in a nursing home?

12. Will the family be able to pull closer together around the nursing home placement?

13. Have physicians and other professionals recommended such a placement?

14. Have the caregiver's approaches to daily problems become ineffective?

Dementia is common in nursing homes.
Nursing homes are becoming more aware of the needs of the Alzheimer's patient and the family. Nursing homes have been dealing with this illness disguised by other names for a very long

time, and a high percentage of the persons in nursing homes have some form of dementia or cognitive impairment.

Determine whether the Alzheimer's unit provides special services. Some nursing homes have developed Alzheimer's units to more adequately address the total care needs of these individuals, and others are considering such approaches. Special Alzheimer's programs can provide a more meaningful role for family members. However, families must determine whether such units actually provide specialized services rather than just grouping the patients together.

When choosing a nursing home for a relative with Alzheimer's disease, families should consider several factors.

1. Is the staff physician familiar with Alzheimer's?
2. Are staff at all levels of the nursing home aware of the needs and problems associated with this disease (e.g., administrative, nursing, dietary, and activities staff)?
3. How do staff interact with residents who are similarly impaired?
4. What activities are provided for persons with Alzheimer's and other dementias?
5. Is the physical plant of the facility well organized, attractive, and designed to encourage either socialization or privacy as appropriate?
6. Does the facility encourage family involvement and support groups?
7. Is the atmosphere friendly?
8. What provisions are made to prevent wandering?
9. Is the building particularly noisy?
10. Is there a safe area for the person to walk outside?
11. How does the facility deal with residents who are noisy and hard to manage?
12. How are drugs and restraints used in behavior management?
13. Is the facility a reasonable distance from your home?

14. Do Alzheimer's units utilize a special approach to needs of these residents?

Some families may realize that a nursing home may be the most appropriate resource for the care of their relatives with Alzheimer's disease. Still, they may have built barriers to seeking the placement. Some concerns are practical, others psychological. The following example illustrates some psychological barriers that should be overcome.

Suzy was the middle-aged daughter of a 75-year-old man who had Alzheimer's disease. Suzy was the primary caregiver because her two brothers lived out of town. Her relationship with her father had not been particularly close. However, she shouldered the responsibility for his care, partly because she felt guilty about her past with her family. She had been divorced for ten years, and during that time she had assumed a major role in caring for her parents. She still believed her brothers should help more, but their explanations for not being more involved generally were reasonable. They did help somewhat with financial needs. Her mother had died a year before in a nursing home. Now her father was living with her.

The mother had a strong role in caring for Suzy's father until she had suffered a stroke, which eventually precipitated her placement in the nursing home. At that time, the father had objected to his wife's leaving. Suzy thought he had been angry with her since that time; certainly he was more agitated. Suzy had visited her mother in the nursing home, taking her father along. These visits had often upset her father. He would accuse her of trying to put him away.

Now the father required more care and supervision. Suzy still felt some guilt about the past, but she experienced new feelings of guilt about her mother's placement and how she thought it had affected her father. She was experiencing more guilt in caring for her father. It was painful to Suzy when he asked for his wife or called Suzy by his wife's name. One night he talked frequently about going home. Suzy did her best to assure him he was home, but in his state of agitation, he would not listen. Later that night he wandered from the house.

Suzy's father was not found until the early morning hours by the police, who took him to a hospital emergency room. Suzy was awakened by a call after her name and number were found in his billfold. Her dad was so confused and agitated that he had to be placed in a psychiatric hospital for a few days.

The father responded well to that setting, yet it appeared to the hospital staff that he needed more care than Suzy could provide at home. Nursing home placement was recommended, but Suzy insisted that she must care for him at home. For a while her position seemed unreasonable to staff until the past and current sources of guilt were uncovered. Suzy actually believed she could provide better care in her home, particularly now that her dad was more stable.

Hospital staff agreed to support this decision if Suzy would get help from some community services to help her manage her father and deal with her needs. Counseling eventually helped Suzy to accept her limitations in caring for her father. She finally reconciled her feelings of guilt to the extent that she was willing to look at some other nursing homes. She had gotten involved in the Alzheimer's Family Support Group whose members helped her look at some facilities better equipped to care for Alzheimer's patients and to involve family members in constructive ways. Suzy also involved her brothers in the decision, so she did not have to feel it was her decision alone.

Three months later the placement was made. After a month, Suzy was confident they had made the right decision when she saw her father doing a little better than he had at home. She became involved in some of the nursing home's activities and maintained a modified caregiving role with her father. She began to have a life of her own again.

Finances can be a real barrier to nursing home care. Financial arrangements can be a practical barrier to nursing home placements even when families desire placement. Public assistance programs for nursing homes, such as Medicaid, have financial requirements that must be fulfilled before the cost is covered by a mixture of state and federal funding. Family members should investigate this resource long before their relative needs nursing home care. Too often nursing home placement is sought in a crisis. A hospital may be about to discharge the person, or the caregiver may either have become too ill or too overwhelmed to continue to provide care himself.

In many states—Texas for one—there are two types of eligibility that must be met before nursing home placement can be covered by state and federal financial resources: financial and medical. This can be confusing to families. Not only are there two types of eligibility, but there are also two different state departments that approve the two types of eligibility. Since Alzheimer's disease is not yet uniformly considered a medical condition, there may be problems in getting medical eligibility established. The deficits in the person's functioning must be almost overemphasized for the person to qualify as having medical and nursing care needs. The treating physician may not be familiar with all aspects of daily functioning and mental status. (Forms in the appendix should be helpful in establishing the degree of impairment.)

Families may need to elicit help from attorneys and other agencies in establishing financial and medical eligibility. Private pay does not require such planning, but many people with Alzheimer's disease cannot afford private pay at all. Contact with nursing homes may help families seeking nursing home placement if they start making their plans early. Agencies involved in establishing eligibility should be contacted to determine what information is required. Steps in that process should be fully understood by families. As a rule, if families are familiar with eligibility requirements and the process involved in nursing home care, the eventual placement will take place more smoothly. Early planning also enables family members, particularly the spouse who remains at home, a chance to plan for financial security.

Some patients with Alzheimer's disease may be eligible for other long-term care services, such as placement at a Veteran's Administration (VA) hospital or nursing home care unit. This too should be investigated so that family expectations can be based on facts and not assumptions. The placement may not be possible because the veteran does not meet eligibility requirements. Others who meet requirements may not stay in the VA system for long-term care. The VA also contracts with community nursing homes for placement.

Changes Affecting Nursing Home Placement

States have been implementing new policies and procedures that concern the placement of certain individuals in nursing homes. These changes have resulted from extensive and far-reaching revisions of federal laws that govern nursing home care and Medicaid eligibility. One result of Omnibus Budget Reconciliation Act of 1987 (OBRA) is a more careful screening of persons entering nursing homes (PASARR). A degree of screening for medical eligibility has always been required for admission into a nursing home that receives federal funding. The purpose of the PASARR screening process is the determination of the presence of mental retardation or mental illness in persons seeking nursing home care. This prevents persons with these conditions from being inappropriately placed in nursing homes.

Individuals who are either mentally retarded or who experience more intense manifestations of mental illness may be excluded from nursing home placement. Those that need nursing home care may be required to have specialized treatments, training, and other services before they can enter a nursing home. Persons already in nursing homes are evaluated regularly to determine if their conditions warrant intervention. For example, a resident who has become extremely psychotic and difficult to manage may be found to need more "active" psychiatric treatment. If the degree of needed treatment cannot be provided in the nursing home, psychiatric hospitalization may be indicated.

Everyone seeking admission into a nursing home receiving federal funding must be screened, whether paying privately or needing Medicaid. The new laws are meant to prevent inappropriate placement of individuals in nursing homes. Presumably persons in nursing homes who need psychiatric services will have these needs addressed. The mentally retarded and other persons with developmental disabilities or conditions will receive the services they need. If the screening process excludes these individuals from entering a nursing home, caregivers will be responsible for finding ways to address their needs in the community.

Alzheimer's excluded   Fortunately the advocacy of many people and groups has ensured that persons with Alzheimer's or other related disorders have been excluded from diagnostic categories that indicate mental illness and the contingent need for psychiatric treatment. However, when it becomes necessary to consider nursing home placement, Alzheimer's families can prevent some unnecessary problems that can be associated with the PASARR screening.

The diagnosis must reflect an appropriate work-up. Neurological, medical, and even neuropsychological evaluations may be necessary to document the nature and extent of impairment that cannot be attributed to other causes. Diagnostics that are based on superficial and incomplete evaluations may not be accepted by the preliminary

PASARR screening. Some persons have been carelessly diagnosed so that a nursing home placement would be possible. Alzheimer's must be the *primary* diagnosis.

Psychiatric medications are used to manage specific symptoms associated with Alzheimer's disease, for example, agitation, delusions and hallucinations, anxiety, and sleeping problems. Antidepressants are used to treat the depression that is secondary to Alzheimer's and a source of excess disability. Medical and psychiatric reports must indicate the rationale for prescribed medications, and the symptoms that are specifically addressed by the medications.

Depression or other psychiatric disorders can accompany Alzheimer's disease. These disorders may have been diagnosed before the Alzheimer's diagnosis was finally made. Although Alzheimer's disease is excluded from the PASARR screening, depression and psychiatric disorders that have psychotic symptoms are not. Psychiatric medications may be given for symptom management of the other psychiatric disorders, for example, bipolar or schizoaffective disorders. A diagnosis of Alzheimer's may be "suspect" when other psychiatric disorders have been a part of the individual's medical history. When other disorders like these or depression are present, it is best to be sure they are listed as secondary diagnoses.

OBRA as a barrier to appropriate care
The inappropriate use of psychiatric medications in nursing homes will be reduced some by the revised nursing home laws (OBRA). Nursing homes seem to be reluctant to support the appropriate use of these medications when behavioral and environmental management strategies are unsuccessful in the management of difficult symptoms. This may create a new dilemma for families who have placed a loved one with Alzheimer's disease in a nursing home. Rather than appropriate psychiatric treatment being implemented, the facility may request that the family move the patient. OBRA has also strengthened the "rights" of nursing home patients, but the facility may be well within its rights in requiring families to move loved ones.

If family caregivers have any questions about how the screening process, or nursing home placement will affect the care of their loved one, they need to seek professional help from the individuals and agencies involved in the PASARR process. Area Agencies on Aging, Ombudsman Programs, and nursing home personnel can direct you to the appropriate help when it is not within the scope of their services.

Final Resource Considerations

Family members caring for a relative with Alzheimer's disease usually have more resources and services available to them than they utilize. Long-term care in the home is possible. In some cases care can be provided in the home until the relative's death. Planning care will involve the need for strategic utilization of community resources, other family members, and friends. Services for Alzheimer's care vary from one community to the next. Rural areas and small towns usually have fewer services than urban areas.

Costs for services also vary. Some have state, federal, and local funding. Others are funded by foundations and other grant sources. Still others are private and require full payment unless other arrangements can be made. Insurance may cover some services, but at this point family members should not assume too much about insurance coverage. They should investigate what types of care and services insurance will cover and for how long. Some families face a difficult predicament when they assume insurance covers nursing home care. While policies may cover some nursing home care, long-term care is not usually covered.

Few communities have sufficient and affordable resources for Alzheimer's care, particularly day care alternatives and respite care services. Other services may be unavailable or simply inadequate to meet the ongoing needs of in-home care. Many provider-type programs that supply in-home services such as cleaning and personal care cannot accept responsibility for supervision. The hours a week that such services can be provided are often limited. In-home supervision is, nevertheless, a major need. On a short-term basis, in-home respite care or a brief respite placement can be beneficial.

Persons living alone and suspected of having an Alzheimer's-type condition are quite difficult to help when family is absent or nonexistent. In these cases some type of guardianship or protective services may be necessary to provide care. Unfortunately, many communities do not have guardianship programs where a nonrelative guardian can be appointed. Mental health authorities may be able to help if these persons reach a point where they are a danger to themselves or others. However, even then the long-range plans may have no solutions.

Family caregivers are a source of ideas for what services are needed in their communities. In fact, families feel less helpless in these situations when they find a way to bring needs to the attention of agencies and others who develop programs in the community. One of the better options is to contact an Area Agency on Aging, which is charged with the responsibility of identifying needs of the elderly, planning for those needs, implementing, and monitoring programs funded under the Older Americans Act. (See the list of these agencies in the appendix.) There may also be other community agencies which are active in planning and program development. The Area Agency on Aging may be able to direct caregivers to these other resources in the community.

ENIGMA

Isn't it strange . . .
That which we have long perceived
as a burden—
the care of a sick loved one—
the care that went on
and on and on—is over now?

It was tiring, and confining,
and discouraging and demeaning at times.
Yet—in a strange way—
I can feel no relief.

Perhaps, inadvertently,
he gave my life a purpose—
a purpose I hardly recognized
nor appreciated.

Now I need a new purpose
(and I am old for that).
That covenant has been kept
as best I knew how—
But my life goes on.

Help me to find a new purpose—
a new resolve—
and let it be a life that doesn't
just keep on living.

Maude S. Newton

PART II

RESEARCH AND TREATMENT

In this part of the book, we have dealt with the more technical aspects of Alzheimer's disease, first describing the physiology of the brain and the changes that take place, then discussing treatment possibilities, keeping in mind that developments are happening daily. Finally, we describe medications typically used and possible side effects.

SURVIVORS

For years I've watched
an old mesquite tree—
gnarled and bent and twisted—
buffeted by winds and droughts.

It starts to grow up
toward the sun and sky.
But the soil is so poor,
the water so scarce,
the heat so fierce,
so cold at times,
it was beat to the ground.

Each Winter you'd think,
—It's dead, for sure!
It's succumbed to the odds
stacked against it.

Yet wait 'til the Spring
and a miracle occurs,
New life springs up
from the gnarled old branches—
a tiny chartreuse sprout
heads straight for the sun!
It lives—overcoming
all that is hard,
telling all the world,
—I live, I will survive!

Sometimes I feel like that old mesquite tree
I feel battered by life's adversities,
I feel down—but not out!
When Spring rolls around,
I feel a fresh stirring of life.

I have things to do—
places I want to explore,
people I love!
I can hold my head high—
look the world in the eye—
and say,
—I live, I will survive!

Maude S. Newton

14

ABNORMAL CHANGES IN
THE BRAIN

For hundreds of years, the symptoms of what we now know as Alzheimer's disease were attributed to senility and old age, or perhaps in more recent times they were attributed to hardening of the arteries and psychosis. In the past, people feared that one day just because they were old, they would "go crazy," lose their memory, and become completely helpless without ever knowing why. With the identification of Alzheimer's disease, however, it has become possible to properly diagnose persons suffering from this illness and to at least partially alleviate their suffering. The next step, at which medical researchers currently are at work, is to isolate the exact biological causes of the disease. Once these causes are known, we can begin to develop effective treatments for Alzheimer's and perhaps someday even find a complete cure.

The next two chapters of this book offer a look at the research done to date on both the causes and treatment of Alzheimer's. This research has revealed physical and chemical changes present in brains affected by Alzheimer's, suggested possible causes of the disease, and included experiments with promising treatments.

Because the research completed leaves many questions unanswered, most of the material covered here must remain somewhat speculative. Although a great deal has been learned to date, no definiive answer to the mysteries posed by Alzheimer's disease has been found. The research findings are valuable, however, because they allow caregivers to understand more fully the changes occurring within the Alzheimer's patient. In addition, the very real progress made gives hope that someday—we all hope soon—medical research will lead us to a clear-cut strategy for the disease's treatment and prevention.

The final chapter covers the use of current medications used in treating some of the psychiatric manifestations of Alzheimer's disease. Agitation, anxiety, delusions, and sleeping difficulties present behavior management problems to family caregivers. Careful use of psychiatric medications can make caregiving much easier.

Physical Changes in the Brain

Abnormalities are found in the brains of Alzheimer's patients.

When a person is diagnosed as having Alzheimer's disease, the brain has already deteriorated to some degree. Almost without exception, physical abnormalities (such as neurofibrillary tangles, neuritic plaques, and others) are present in the cerebral cortex, the outer layer of the brain that governs such higher functions as memory, thinking, and reasoning.

Several of the abnormal characteristics of brains affected by Alzheimer's disease are associated with the most basic and important part of the brain, the neurons (also called nerve cells). The brain consists of many billions of neurons, which are its means of receiving and sending messages. Neurons can be viewed as the way different parts of the brain communicate with each other and the rest of the body. One neuron of the brain may communicate with as many as 1000 other neurons although these units of communication usually send messages to only a few neurons. Alzheimer's disease is somehow responsible for a loss of neurons. Some of the physical abnormalities, for example, neurofibrillary tangles, occur in the body of neurons. These changes might contribute to destruction of nerve cells or compromise their functioning.

Connection between disease and abnormalities

Because the tangles, plaques, and other physical abnormalities so consistently accompany the disease, researchers feel certain that some connection exists between these brain abnormalities and the mental and emotional changes that Alzheimer's patients experience. What is not well known is whether these physical changes are directly related to the cause of Alzheimer's disease or whether other aspects of the disease itself cause the abnormalities. In the latter, the physical changes would be manifestations of the illness. These are questions future research will continue to address.

Connections between abnormalities and impairments
We do know that a direct correlation exists between the degree and the distribution of physical abnormalities and the severity of Alzheimer's-type dementia. We also know that the abnormalities discussed in this chapter tend to be concentrated in areas of the brain that control abilities most affected by Alzheimer's. These findings suggest that physical changes in the brain make some contribution to the disease's impairments.

Anatomy of the Brain

To understand how Alzheimer's affects the brain, we first must understand the basics of brain anatomy and the ways in which various areas of the brain are related to specific mental functions.

Brain's cortex
The outer surface of the brain is known as the cerebral cortex (see Figure 1). Accounting for about 80 percent of total brain mass, the cortex is divided into two nearly symmetrical hemispheres: the left and the right. Each of these hemispheres is divided in turn into four lobes: the frontal, the parietal, the temporal, and the occipital.

Frontal lobes
The frontal lobes mediate motor functions, govern emotional behavior, help organize sequential physical movements, determine some abilities of expressive speech, and influence personalities, inhibitions, and social behavior. As Alzheimer's disease affects this area of the brain, patients undergo a variety of personality changes, lose inhibitions, and become less able to organize behavior. With damage to the frontal lobes of the brain, persons do not recognize their errors.

Parietal lobes
The parietal lobes are concerned with sensory functions such as physical sensations, touch, and spatial relationships. They also allow us to

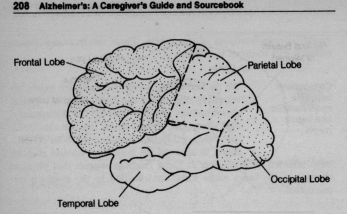

Figure 1. The Cerebral Cortex. The lobes of the brain's cortex. The frontal lobe is at the front of the head. This is a side view of the left hemisphere. The right hemisphere is basically a mirror reflection of the left hemisphere.

recognize patterns in our experience, perform intellectual tasks such as mathematics, and maintain our physical orientation. Disorientation to places can result from damage to this brain area. When Alzheimer's strikes the parietal lobes, patients experience trouble with coordinated, purposeful movements, spatial perceptions, and recognition, among other functions.

Occipital lobes The occipital lobes are the brain's visual center, controlling very basic visual perceptions and bringing together the parts of visual information into a meaningful whole. Damage to this area can lead to loss of the visual field and problems in space perception.

Temporal lobes The temporal lobes are involved in a range of important functions, including hearing, memory, vision, and verbal comprehension. In conjunction with the brain's limbic system, these lobes also affect the experience and memory of emotions such as fear, jealousy, anger, or happiness. Our sense of time and individuality also seems to be located in these

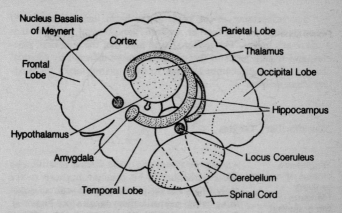

Figure 2.   Brain Areas Affected by Alzheimer's Disease.   This picture of the brain shows areas impacted by Alzheimer's disease abnormalities. The location of the nucleus Basalis of Meynert is an approximation. Other parts of the brain have been omitted because they are not relevant to our discussion. Some parts of the limbic system—the hippocampus, amydala, thalamus, and hypothalamus—are indicated.

lobes (Restak 1984). Of the four brain areas, the temporal lobes appear to be the area most severely affected by Alzheimer's disease. Memory problems, auditory perception, musical perception, difficulties in comprehension, and difficulties in execution of speech all appear to be connected with damage in this area. Problems in focused attention also can be attributed to damage in the temporal lobes.

The limbic system of the brain affects memory and emotions.

Enveloped by the cortex are a number of other brain areas relevant to an understanding of Alzheimer's disease. Some of these are part of the limbic system, a group of brain structures which have influence on our emotions and behavior. The parts of the limbic system most involved in the damage associated with Alzheimer's disease include the amygdala, believed to affect emotion, and the hippocampus, believed to affect both short-term and long-term memory (see Figure 2).

The importance of the parts of the brain just described will become clear as we further explore the physical changes that Alzheimer's brings. The reader should note that the temporal, parietal, and frontal lobes of the cortex are more affected by physical changes. The hippocampus seems to be a prime target for physical abnormalities.

Neurofibrillary Tangles

Tangles are clumps of ordinary filaments in the brain that have become abnormally twisted.

Among the symptoms of the disease identified by Alois Alzheimer in his original diagnosis in the early 1900s was the presence in the brain of something called neurofibrillary tangles (see Figure 3). Simply put, neurofibrillary tangles are bundles of ordinary brain filaments that have become badly twisted. When such tangles are viewed under an electron microscope, one can see little hair-like structures called filaments. When these filaments occur in pairs, they are wrapped around each other in a spiral fashion (Reisberg 1981), somewhat like two pieces of yarn that have been twisted together and then stretched tightly. These paired filaments are known as paired helical filaments, a term sometimes used to refer to neurofibrillary tangles. Filaments are normal; they become abnormal when their form is changed by twisting.

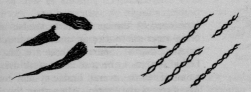

Figure 3. Neurofibrillary Tangles and Paired Helical Filaments.   If the image of tangles to the left were enlarged, lines would take the appearance of the paired helical filaments to the right.

All older people develop some tangles in those parts of the brain that affect memory and behavior.

Interestingly, some degree of neurofibrillary tangle formation is found in virtually all examined brain tissue of persons over age 90 (Reisberg 1981). Tangles also are found in specific brain areas of most normal middle-aged and older persons. When their brain tissue is examined microscopically, tangle formations are particularly evident in the hippocampus, the area that plays a role in both recent memory functions and the storage and retrieval of long-term memory (Beaumont 1983). It has some involvement in learning. The hippocampus further seems to be involved in bringing together various forms of incoming sensory information (Bloom et al. 1985), the inhibition of responses, the organization of movement, and spatial organization (Kolb and Whishaw 1980). Another area where concentrations of tangles are found is the amygdala, which has a role in fear reactions and aggressive behavior. It is also suspected of having some role in memory with the hippocampus. The reader will recall that both of these structures are part of the brain's limbic system, which has a major role in expression and experience of emotion (Kolb and Whishaw 1980).

The more severe problems with memory and behavior associated with Alzheimer's may be caused by more severe problems with tangles.

Since aging persons tend to exhibit a high incidence of tangles in brain areas associated with memory as well as memory problems, it seems possible that the development of slight short-term memory loss with age could be associated with subtle damage to the hippocampus. It further follows that the more severe memory disorders of Alzheimer's patients as well as related problems might be associated with more severe hippocampal damage. Similarly, the lack of emotional response to memory problems found early in Alzheimer's, sometimes called a blunted or flat effect, could be associated with damage to the amygdala, while damage to the overall limbic system could account for patients' loss of emotional control. Altogether, the damage caused by tangles to these parts of the brain could be responsible for some of the emotional disturbances and personality changes exhibited by Alzheimer's victims.

Because tangles appear to occur naturally with age, the mere presence of tangles in the brain does not indicate disease. What is different about the brains of Alzheimer's patients, however, is the location and number of tangles. In Alzheimer's victims, tangles tend to be significantly concentrated in the hippocampus and in far higher numbers than in the brains of normal aging persons. They also are concentrated in the cerebral cortex, particularly in the parietal-temporal region and the association cortex. The association areas of the cortex bring together information from the areas around which they are located. It is in these areas that the brain integrates immediate sensory information with memories and emotions, thus making it possible for us to think, decide, and plan behavior. Since such integrated thought typically becomes difficult for Alzheimer's patients, the damage observed in the association cortex seems particularly significant.

Other small but important areas of the brain are affected by neurofibrillary tangles. These small areas represent collections of nerve cells that serve as stimulation centers for neurons ascending into the brain's cortex. Neurons or brain cells of the brain comprise an intricate network through which information can be transmitted and received.

Groups of neurons within the brain's network are specifically adapted to communicate with their own chemical messenger which is called a neurotransmitter. These special networks of neurotransmitters, specific nerve cells, each receive stimulation from their own collection of nerve cells deeper in the brain. For example, for the neurotransmitter acetylcholine which is deficient in the Alzheimer's brain, the source of stimulation is called the nucleus basalis of Meynert (see Figure 2). This brain area has a significant concentration of tangles.

Tangles are also found in the localized areas of the brain that act as stimulation centers for neurons using the neurotransmitters norepinephrine, serotonin, and dopamine (Bondareff 1986). Chemical changes in the brain are discussed later in this chapter.

Research has shown that the larger the number of tangles found in Alzheimer's patients, the greater the degree of dementia.

The correlations discovered make it likely that tangles are directly linked to the impairment of brain function, though research has not yet uncovered precisely what that link might be. Some research suggests that tangles may have some role in neuronal deterioration and destruction. The loss of neurons may also be secondary to other unknown aspects of the disease process. Other research has shown that the larger the number of tangles found, along with another abnormality known as senile plaques, the higher is the degree of dementia observed in Alzheimer's victims. This further confirms the suspicion that tangles and plaques may be a source of the disease's impairments.

Other dementing illnesses are also associated with tangles.

As an interesting sidelight, neurofibrillary tangles also have been found in other types of dementing illnesses. Among these are dementia pugilistica (punch-drunkenness), a dementia observed in veteran boxers; the rare Parkinsonian-dementia complex of Guam (Reisberg 1981); post-encephalitic Parkinson's disease (Bondareff 1986); and other forms of infectious dementias. Another disorder in which tangles are very frequently present is Down's syndrome, the genetic abnormality that causes mental retardation. Persons with Down's syndrome who live past age 40 invariably develop tangles, plaques, and other pathological changes common to Alzheimer's disease (Katzmann 1986), and the tangles are similarly located in the brain (Reisberg 1981).

Current research on neurofibrillary tangles focuses on unlocking the composition and abnormal protein source of the paired helical filaments. This is important because the protein in paired helical filaments is not common to the brain. Some researchers suggest that since the protein might come from a source external to the brain, an unconventional virus may be implicated (Selkoe 1987). Paired helical filaments have also been found in neuritic plaques. Further investigation of the paired helical filaments may lead to other clues to the cause(s) of Alzheimer's disease because they have not been found in the brains of neurologically normal persons (Davies and Wolozin 1987). By learning more about tangles, it is hoped that we will also uncover significant answers about the causes of Alzheimer's disease.

Senile or Neuritic Plaques

Significance of plaques   Like neurofibrillary tangles, plaques were among the physical abnormalities noticed by Alois Alzheimer in his original diagnosis of the disease. As with tangles, plaques are found in the brains of normal aged persons; however, they appear in far more significant concentrations in the brains of Alzheimer's victims, appear in those parts of the brain that are most affected by the disease, and are most prevalent in the most severely affected individuals. In fact, plaques appear to be an even better indicator of the degree of dementia than do neurofibrillary tangles.

Types of plaques and description   There are three types of plaques: primitive, classical, and amyloid. Classical and amyloid plaques both contain more amyloid. All types of plaques can be found in Alzheimer's disease. In classical plaques the amyloid is contained by the core; amyloid plaques consist almost entirely of this amyloid material (Wisniewski 1983). The classical plaque is easier to picture (see Figure 4). There is the central core of amyloid that appears fuzzy and fibrous. This core is surrounded by a ring of degenerating fragments of cells which resemble a loosely-arranged crown of thorns. The fragments are like the debris of brain cells and include axons, dendrites, and slender filaments. Paired helical filaments of neurofibrillary tangles can be found in the debris around the classical plaque's core. Neuritic or senile plaques are the more general terms used for the three types of plaques.

Plaques are found outside neurons, whereas neurofibrillary tangles are found in neurons. In Alzheimer's disease, plaques are abnormal, particularly because they occur more frequently than in the brains of normal aged persons. Plaques also occur in other diseases of the brain.

Locations of plaques   As with tangles, plaques tend to be more abundant in the cerebral cortex and are found in smaller numbers in other parts of the brain such

Figure 4.   Classical Neuritic Plaque.   The primitive plaque consists mainly
of the clustered debris outside the core of this plaque. Amyloid plaques consist
of the core material of the plaque.

as the thalamus. Rarely, they have been found in the cerebellum
(Bondareff 1986). The thalamus receives sensory information and has
some control of our motor activity. It helps us be generally aware of
touch, temperature, and pain. the cerebellum primarily coordinates
muscular activity and receives information from other parts of the
body such as skin, muscles, and joints.

Some indication of damage to the thalamus may be observed
during the course of Alzheimer's disease. Damage associated with
the cerebellum would be more difficult to observe until perhaps the
later stages of the illness. Functions assigned to the hippocampus and
cortex are more easily recognized and more severely disturbed. Memory impairment and disturbances in thinking, judgment, and speech
are common features of Alzheimer's disease.

**Amyloid and
plaques**

With regard to this disease, the significance of
plaques rests not only on their concentration in
areas of the brain that are most impaired, but the
presence of amyloid is also important. Amyloid
is a part of the plaques, and research has shown enduring interest in
amyloid because it is thought that understanding this abnormal protein might yield clues to Alzheimer's cause.

**Amyloid and
disease**

Amyloid has been associated with a variety of
diseases that include turberculosis, Hodgkin's
disease, and cancer. Such severe neurological illnesses as Creutzfeldt-Jakob disease and Kuru are assoicated with ac-
cumulations of amyloid. Both are caused by slow viruses.

Amyloid and the immune system

Amyloid is known to be deposited in tissues which experience altered immunity (Thienhaus et al. 1985). For some reason, the body's immune system does not protect the body from disease effectively. The possibility is raised that Alzheimer's disease might result from breakdown in the body's immune system. Instead of protecting the brain, the immune system turns on the brain. This suggests an autoimmune response whereby the body produces antibodies that are directed against its own healthy tissue. The immune system cannot tell the difference between normal and foreign substances.

Amyloid and prions

The understanding of amyloid has been advanced some by the work of Prusiner and his coworkers. Amyloid plaques were found in a slow virus disease (scrapie) in sheep and goats. This disease has been transmitted to a hamster brain. The brain tissue was found to contain very small rod-shaped particles called prions. Prions are protein-like infectious particles (Goldsmith 1984) which are smaller than a virus. In a certain configuration prions have a remarkable resemblance to amyloid plaques, causing some researchers to hope that amyloid plaques may be found to be associated with prions. This would provide some evidence that a similar slow virus might cause Alzheimer's disease. However, the amyloid plaque in this disease could also be formed from proteins other than prions. The issue of what causes amyloid in plaques has not been settled.

Down's syndrome

The significance of neuritic plaques has been examined from another perspective. The amyloid proteins found in Alzheimer's disease are thought to be the same amyloid present in Down's syndrome (Davies and Wolozin 1987). In the Down's syndrome brain, neuritic plaques containing amyloid (as well as other abnormalities associated with Alzheimer's) typically appear in abundance and are distributed in much the same way as in Alzheimer's disease. Down's syndrome is characterized by extra copies of chromosome 21 and is a genetic disorder.

Chromosome 21 and Alzheimer's

In 1987 some significant findings occurred involving chromosome 21 and Alzheimer's disease. An abnormal gene on this chromosome shows a genetic defect that is thought to be responsible for a familial form of Alzheimer's disease. This indicates that some cases of Alzheimer's disease are under genetic control. This same chromosome contains a gene that is responsible for producing a major protein component of amyloid. The gene is now known as the amyloid precursor protein (APP). It is the parent protein of the smaller chain of amino acids that comprise the protein fragment beta amyloid.

Amyloid in Down's syndrome

The APP gene might account for more beta amyloid in the Down's syndrome brain. Since there are extra copies of chromosome 21 in this disorder, there would be more copies of the gene influencing the production of amyloid. This line of reasoning, however, cannot explain amyloid in Alzheimer's disease because there is no duplication of the amyloid gene.

Amyloid mystery

Aging itself may be a factor. As we age, amyloid may be produced. This could explain why Alzheimer's disease increases in older persons. We know that amyloid is present in the walls of cerebral vessels of aged persons (Wisniewski 1978). However, even with these deposits of amyloid, plaques do not necessarily occur. It is not clear if vascular amyloid, which is fairly common in both Alzheimer's disease and old age, has the same origin and chemical composition as the amyloid in plaques. Amyloid's presence in plaques remains a puzzle.

Amyloid near cause of Alzheimer's

At present, we only know that amyloid plays a central role in Alzheimer's disease. We do not know how. It may very well be closely connected either with the cause of Alzheimer's disease or with other underlying conditions that will lead to the cause. Since it now appears that every person has a gene that plays a part in the production of amyloid, we must question why everyone does not get Alzheimer's disease. Researchers suspect that some other factor or factors must combine with the amyloid gene's role in order for

Alzheimer's disease to develop. These factors might be a virus, some chemical extraneous to the brain or body, immune system break-down, or factors that simply have not been identified.

Amyloid in plaques common in Alzheimer's disease raises many questions for research. Our understanding of amyloid is growing. It is associated with plaques, tangles, and cerebral vessels. We also know that the brain's loss of neurons corresponds with the distribution of plaques and tangles. Tangles and plaques particularly are indicators of the severity of dementia. The greater the concentration of plaques, the greater is the impairment of brain function. We cannot yet say that plaques cause the loss of brain cells.

Amyloid may act with other as yet unidentified factors in Alzheimer's disease which accelerate the production of amyloid. As a result of this, interaction in offensive proteins may be changed into harmful deposits of amyloids. Science may be able to discover ways to frustrate the genetic production of amyloid. Other factors must be identified that can explain why everyone who has an amyloid gene does not develop Alzheimer's disease.

Other protein abnormalities   Since cells are comprised of proteins, researchers have become interested in abnormal proteins. Other proteins act as conduits for chemical messengers. Two of these, tau protein and MAP (microtubule-associated protein), are found in increased amounts of abnormal forms in some victims of Alzheimer's disease (Mace and Rabins 1991). According to the theory about these protein abnormalities, the body may not be able to break them down. As a result, abnormal proteins accumulate in the brain.

Granulovacuolar Degeneration

Description of GVD   A third type of brain abnormality, granulovacuolar degeneration (GVD), has an attraction to neurons in the hippocampus of the Alzheimer's victim's brain. GVD strikes the area of brain cells around their nucleus (see Figure 5), the area called cytoplasm. One or more fluid-filled spaces, vacuoles, form in the cell's cytoplasm with GVD. Within the vacuoles there is a dense, granular material (Ball 1983) which under an electron microscope appears to have a crystalline

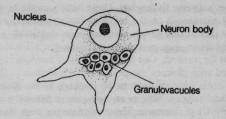

Figure 5. Granulovacuolar Degeneration in a Neuron. Note that numerous granulovacuoles have formed in the body of this neuron around the nucleus.

structure (Conley 1987). As these granulovacuoles develop, they cause a swelling of the cell's cytoplasm which may eventually lead to degeneration or dysfunction of the brain cell itself.

GVD and normal aging   With normal aging, GVD also appears in the hippocampal area, but its concentration and severity are relatively low, and this degeneration occurs at a relatively slow rate with aging (Kemper 1984). The rate of GVD is more rapid in Alzheimer's disease. Neurofibrillary tangles are also prevalent in the hippocampal area where high concentrations of GVD are found in Alzheimer's disease.

GVD and memory impairment. Occurs in diminished hippocampal cells   The severity of impaired memory functions associated with the hippocampus in Alzheimer's disease can be more fully appreciated when one considers that GVD occurs within an already shrinking population of neurons. More than one-half of the original neurons of the hippocampus may have been lost, which is suspected to be up to five times more serious than cell loss in normal aging (Ball 1983). Both GVD and tangles occur in this diminished cell population.

Role of hippocampus   The hippocampus is commonly given a major role in memory functions. Cells in the rear portion of the hippocampus, an area thought to be more involved in remote memories, are especially vulnerable to GVD. It thus appears that GVD may contribute to the disruption of more remote memories, a type of memory impairment that is most evident in later stages of Alzheimer's disease.

Future research and GVD

Though much remains to be discovered about GVD, some researchers believe it may have an even stronger relationship with certain types of behavioral deterioration than plaques and tangles (Ball 1983). This contention requires more investigation. Because GVD and tangles are closely matched in respect to their occurrence and location in the hippocampus, the possibility of related causes for both has been considered (Reisberg 1983). GVD was first described as a characteristic of dementia in 1911, but investigation of this abnormality in Alzheimer's disease is relatively recent. For that reason it has not received the attention given to the classic brain abnormalities of Alzheimer's disease, the tangles and plaques.

Hirano Bodies

Description of Hirano bodies

A fourth abnormality of Alzheimer's disease, first described by Hirano in 1965, is known as the Hirano body. This is a discreet type of change primarily seen in the hippocampus. A microscopic spindle-shaped structure (Kemper 1984), a Hirano body resembles a string of red blood cells (Davies and Wolozin 1987). Under an electron microscope, Hirano bodies appear to have a crystalline structure (Brun 1983). Hirano bodies invade the cell body of a neuron and also its processes (axons and dendrites). Neither the nature nor the importance of Hirano bodies has been clearly established although these abnormal structures have been associated with actin (Davies and Wolozin 1987), a major protein found in muscle fibers.

Age-related change

As with other abnormalities typical of Alzheimer's disease, the appearance of Hirano bodies in the brain is an age-related change. The bodies begin to appear in very small numbers during a person's teens, with a significant increase occurring only during and after the 60s. All persons over age 80 have Hirano bodies (Kemper 1984).

Hirano bodies and memory loss

Exactly how Hirano bodies affect the memory functions of the hippocampus is not known. However, some research suggests that Hirano bodies may trap ribosomes, rendering them dormant. Ribosomes are the agents that change RNA molecules—a basic unit of memory—into proteins, allowing the RNA to do its job of forming memories. If Hirano bodies are imprisoning the necessary ribosomes, then they may be preventing RNA from doing its job so that memories are not being formed. Further study testing this theory still is needed.

Congophilic Angiopathy

In this condition, amyloid is found deposited in cerebral blood vessels.

Amyloid, the problematic protein found in senile plaques, also appears deposited abnormally in the walls of cerebral arteries, capillaries, and tiny veins. Because amyloid is a congophilic material (one that picks up a dye known as congo red, used to identify tissues), the presence of these abnormal deposits in blood vessels is called congophilic angiopathy, or simply amyloid angiopathy (angiopathy meaning a disorder of the blood vessels).

Somehow related to Alzheimer's

The significance of congophilic angiopathy has not been clearly established, but there does appear to be some special connection between the deposits and Alzheimer's: while the condition appears in only 9 percent of neurologically normal individuals, it shows up in 92 percent of Alzheimer's patients. It also appears in all victims of Down's syndrome.

Angiopathy and strokes in Alzheimer's disease

We further know that congophilic angiopathy sometimes leads to hemorrhaging and infarction—tissue death caused by the obstruction of blood vessels—in the Alzheimer's brain. Infarction and hemorrhaging in turn can cause strokes, and strokes can result in dementia. Indeed, multi-infarct dementia—a condition resulting from multiple large or small strokes—accounts for about 15 percent of all dementing brain disorders (Reisberg 1981). A combination of multi-infarct dementia and Alzheimer's disease account for some 25 percent of all dementias in later life. Some researchers thus suspect that congophilic angiopathy is a contributing factor to stroke-induced dementia in Alzheimer's disease.

Possible causes of angiopathy

Other researchers theorize that congophilic angiopathy may signal an abnormality of the immune system of the brain or a deterioration of the blood-brain barrier, the special membrane that protects the brain from foreign substances. The deterioration of this barrier could cause both the angiopathy and the greater occurrence of infarcts and hemorrhage found in the Alzheimer's brain due to formation of amyloid deposits in the brain.

Major points

Research has identified five physical abnormalities of the brain—neurofibrillary tangles, senile or neuritic plaques, granulovacuolar degeneration, Hirano bodies, and congophilic angiopathy—that are consistently present in the brains of Alzheimer's patients. All are present in those parts of the brain that control memory and behavior, particularly in the hippocampus. Some of these same abnormalities also are found in other neurological illnesses that cause dementia and in Down's syndrome, which causes mental retardation. The eventual appearance of all of these abnormalities in the brain is an age-related change, and normal aging brains generally show similar changes although in much lower quantities.

No definite facts are known about the link between these observed abnormalities and the cause of Alzheimer's disease. However, because these abnormalities tend to occur in those areas of the brain that control the functions most affected by the disease, and because they might somehow destroy or disable brain cells, researchers believe they may explain much of the mental impairment suffered by Alzheimer's patients. If the breakdown of nerve cells in Alzheimer's disease can be better understood, it might be possible to prevent the degree of cell destruction in this disease. The chemical treatments currently under investigation depend to a large degree on functional nerve cells which decrease as the disease progresses. Research must still determine if the physical abnormalities represent the debris of this disease process, or if they contribute in some way to the destruction of what had been a functional mind.

Chemical Changes in the Brain

Accompanying the physical abnormalities that appear in the Alzheimer's brain are chemical changes: lowered levels of crucial chemicals that the brain requires to record, process, and store information. These chemicals have been found most significantly lowered in the areas of the brain most affected by Alzheimer's, leading researchers to strongly suspect that chemical changes cause some of the disease's impairments.

More about Brain Anatomy

Neurons send messages to and from the various areas of the brain. At the cellular level, the brain is an intricate network of several billion interconnected cells, each equipped to perform a special task. Others included in this network are the billion or so nerve cells called neurons—the building blocks of a complex communication system that relays messages between the various areas of the brain and between the brain and the rest of the body. These messages travel along neuronal pathways. When plenty of healthy neurons are available to form the pathways, the whole communication system—and thus our thought processses themselves and other brain related abilities—can function properly. However, when large numbers of neurons deteriorate

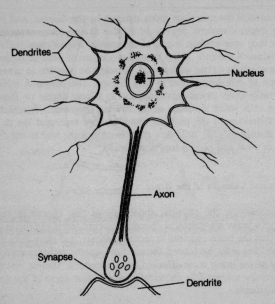

Figure 6. Example of a Neuron from the Brain. Note the axon, which carries the message a neuron sends to the synapse. Neurons have dendrites which receive message from other neurons. (The synapse where the axon and dendrite communicate with a neurotransmitter is enlarged so that the reader can visualize this area.)

or are destroyed, significant disruption of brain function occurs, severely limiting one's ability to think, act, and remember.

Neurons described

Neurons consist of a cell body and nucleus and protrusions called processes which transmit electrochemical messages from one cell to another. One kind of process, called an axon, sends a communication; the other called dendrites receive communications from other neurons (see Figure 6). Each neuron usually has a number

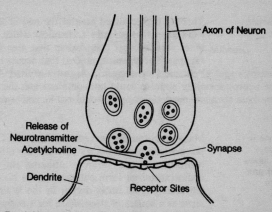

Figure 7. A Neuron's Axon Shown Communicating with a Dendrite of Another Neuron. Neurotransmitter is released into the synapse and picked up at dendrite's receptor sites. The neurotransmitter is made when the enzyme CAT (choline acetyltransferase) combines with acetyl to make acetylcholine, the neurotransmitter of the cholinergic system.

of dendrites (meaning tree with its branches). A remarkable feature of the brain's neurons is the fact that the axons and dendrites link neurons together in circuits. One neuron could conceivably transmit messages to literally hundreds of other neurons. Usually neurons are linked with only a few other recipient neurons. The body of the cell may also have connections with adjoining neurons and receive that neuron's message.

Synapse of a neuron

The actual transmission from an axon to the receiving part of another cell (dendrites or cell body) takes place in the tiny gap between them, called a synapse (see Figure 7). Neurons do not communicate directly by touching each other; the synapse is important because of what happens there. For a message to be conveyed in the special gap (synapse), a chemical message must be transmitted.

Neurotrans-
mitter
There is a specialized area at the end of a neuron's axon that secretes a chemical which combines with another chemical in that area of the
synapse. The chemical process that occurs makes
the neuron's special chemical messenger, a neurotransmitter. Without the neurotransmitter neurons could not communicate; the information these chemical messengers carry would not be conveyed.

Neurons in
pathways
using same
neurotrans-
mitters
Many neurotransmitters exist in the brain. Different neurons in the brain's network use different
neurotransmitters. Neurons utilizing the same
neurotransmitter form pathways in the brain, often arising from areas deeper in the brain that
serve as a source of stimulation for a pathway of
neurons using a common neurotransmitter to send messages. The
neurotransmitter system thought to be involved in thought and memory is called the cholinergic system.

Alzheimer's
disease dis-
ables certain
neurons and
neurotrans-
mitters caus-
ing disruption
of the brain's
communica-
tion system.
In Alzheimer's disease, problems develop in the
brain's communication system. Disturbances or
deficiencies in either the structural mechanisms
(the neurons themselves) or the chemical messengers (the neurotransmitters) can lead to
disturbances in behavior, thought, or emotion.
In particular, Alzheimer's disables the brain's
cholinergic system, which includes the neurotransmitter acetylcholine and its related network
of neurons, known as the cholinergic neurons
(Reisberg 1981) or the cholinergic system.

To a lesser degree the disease may also seem to affect the serotonergic system, which secretes the neurotransmitter serotonin; the
noradrenergic system, which secretes the neurotransmitter noradrenaline (norephinephrine); and the system using the neurotransmitter somatostatin, which is also identified as a neuropeptide. In
this section of the chapter, we will look at the changes wrought by
Alzheimer's disease in each of these important chemical systems and
at the subsequent disturbances in mental function and behavior that
these changes appear to cause.

The Cholinergic System

Cholinergic neurons use the neurotransmitter acetylcholine. From a small area called the nucleus basalis of Meynert, these neurons and their processes reach up and out into the cortex of the brain. When these cholinergic pathways are not functioning, critical messages from one area of the brain to another cannot get through. Thus a healthy cholinergic system—the neurons and their associated chemical messengers—may be essential to our memory, thoughts, judgment, personality, sensory perception, and other higher mental functions. Certainly it is involved in memory and in giving information meaning.

Cholinergic neurons require the neurotransmitter acetylcholine and two enzymes—CAT and AChE—to communicate properly.

Cholinergic neurons communicate by means of a chemical chain reaction, and for the communication to work properly, all of the links in the chain must be in place. To start the process of transmitting information, a neuron secretes in its axon a chemical called acetyl (see Figure 8). The acetyl combines chemically with an enzyme known as choline acetyltransferase (CAT), and the CAT in turn creates the neurotransmitter, acetylcholine, which is released into the synapse. Acetylcholine, carrying its chemical message, is recognized by

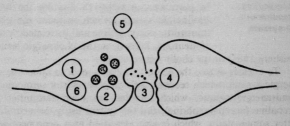

Figure 8.   Neurotransmission.   (1) CAT combines with acetyl, (2) Acetylcholine results, (3) Neurotransmitter released into synapse, (4) Receptors on receiving neuron picks up acetylcholine, (5) Enzyme AchE breaks down acetylcholine, (6) new transmissions begin the process again.

special sites (receptor sites) on the adjoining neuron. The message continues to be transmitted until another enzyme is activated. This enzyme is called acetylcholinesterase (AChE). Without the action of AChE on the acetylcholine, the neuron would be locked in to a message. Other messages could not be sent. Once the message is received by the adjoining cell and the acetylcholine is broken down, the whole process can begin again. It is this simple chemical system that enables the brain's network of neurons to send hundreds of messages throughout the body each minute.

In Alzheimer's disease these vital chemicals are lacking, leading to the destruction of cholinergic neurons.

In Alzheimer's disease, however, this system breaks down. For unknown reasons, the cholinergic neurons begin to lose both their acetylcholine neurotransmitters and the two vital enzymes, CAT and AChE. Research has shown that the cholinergic system in particular is attacked by Alzheimer's disease, and cholinergic neurons are selectively destroyed; however, the cause for this destruction remains puzzling. Also in question is the precise role that the breakdown of this system plays in causing the impairments associated with Alzheimer's disease.

Loss of CAT and AChE associated with impairment

Some research has focused on the loss of the enzymes CAT and AChE, finding that deficiencies of these enzymes tend to accompany physical abnormalities such as plaques and tangles. Cholinergic dysfunction in the hippocampus and in the frontal/parietal areas of the cortex is quite pronounced. Such deficiencies also have been found to correlate with Alzheimer's patients' degree of cognitive impairment and severity of dementia. This suggests that a reduction in enzyme activity alone may impair the cognitive and memory abilities of the whole cholinergic system.

Deficiencies in the enzymes CAT and AChE mean that acetylcholine can neither be made adequately nor effectively broken down again. The cholinergic system's functioning depends heavily on these enzymes carrying out their role effectively.

Origin of cholinergic system and impact of Alzheimer's

Scientists consistently agree that there is a tremendous loss of neurons using acetylcholine in Alzheimer's disease. Now we know that the origin of this system, the nucleus basalis of Meynert, suffers a loss of from 44 to 75 percent of its neurons. This area of the brain is the major source of cholinergic stimulation (Davies and Wolozin 1987; Tagliavini and Pilleri 1983; Coyle et al. 1983). A network of axons from neurons in the nucleus basalis forms cholinergic pathways up to the cortex. The substantial loss of neurons in the origin of cholinergic stimulation will reduce the stimulation to the cortex and hippocampus. Researchers cannot explain why neurons in close proximity to this special nucleus, which do not depend upon acetylcholine, show no significant damage.

When the amount of acetylcholine in the brain is low, patients lose their involvement with life.

Other research has concentrated on the neurotransmitter acetylcholine. This chemical appears to play a unique role in our ability to perceive our environment in a detailed and meaningful way (Restak 1984). It is connected with our ability to become intensely involved in the events around us and to remember what we experience—the appearance of a beautiful garden, perhaps, or the face of a new acquaintance. Conversely, when the amount of acetylcholine diminishes, Alzheimer's patients begin to lose their involvement with and enthusiasm for life. They become detached from the present and drift gradually into the past.

When cholinergic neurons are destroyed, patients suffer memory loss and other cognitive and emotional problems.

Unfortunately, deficiencies in one or more of these associated chemicals may lead to the destruction of the cholinergic neurons themselves. Once large numbers of neurons are damaged, the crucial neuronal pathways leading to and from the frontal/parietal and temporal lobes, the hippocampus, and other brain areas begin to shut down. Damage to the cholinergic pathways in and out of the hippocampus is particularly severe, leaving the hippocampus so isolated from the remainder of the brain that it might as well have been entirely removed (Hyman et al. 1984). This isolation most likely causes severe damage not only to memory functions but also to the patient's emotional health. It also may destroy necessary inhibitions, such as the fear of fire, that were learned through past emotional experience. In sum, damage to the cholinergic pathways linking the hippocampus with the cortex and the limbic structures, including the amygdala, as well as damage to other brain areas, seems to be responsible for much of the emotional and cognitive difficulty experienced by Alzheimer's patients.

The Serotonergic System

A loss of the neurotransmitter serotonin may cause sleep disturbances and mood changes.

Believed to regulate both sleep and sensory perception, the serotonergic system also shows disturbance in Alzheimer's disease. This system relies upon the neurotransmitter serotonin, which is also the chemical thought to induce sleep in the brain. Just as acetylcholine is deficient in the cholinergic system, serotonin has been found significantly reduced in a variety of brain areas when Alzheimer's disease is present (Volicer et al. 1985; Carlsson 1983). Also deficient is serotonin's metabolite (5-HIAA), which is a product of chemical changes related to metabolism. Some research suggests that deficiencies of these two chemicals are related to the sleep disturbances, mood changes, and overly aggressive behavior typical of some Alzheimer's patients (Volicer et al. 1985).

Link with Alzheimer's uncertain

The link between this system and Alzheimer's disease has not yet been as firmly established as the link with the cholinergic system. Current evidence, however, suggests that further research may well uncover important connections between deficiencies in the serotonergic system and Alzheimer's behaviors. For example, some researchers believe that persons with early onsets of dementia may be more likely to have deficiencies in other neurotransmitter systems in addition to the cholinergic system (Mohs et al. 1985).

The Noradrenergic System

Changes in Alzheimer's disease

This system appears to counter the serotonergic system by triggering wakefulness and arousal. Too much of the operative neurotransmitter, noradrenaline, may produce severe stress reactions; too little may cause depression and excessive sleeping. One study reports that noradrenaline is reduced in the Alzheimer's brain by 57 to 74 percent (Gottfries 1985); another indicates that about half of all Alzheimer's patients suffer deficits of noradrenaline in the cortex, with a severe loss in only about 20 percent of that group (Davies and Wolozin 1987). The hippocampus and the hypothalamus also show deficiencies of noradrenaline, of from 49 to 73 percent (Winblad et al. 1982).

A lack of the neurotransmitter noradrenaline may cause emotional and sleep disturbances.

Given the interplay of this system and the serotonergic system, disturbances in either or both neurotransmitters could cause the sleep disturbances found in Alzheimer's disease. Deficits of these chemicals could also explain why some patients become unusually heavily sedated by tranquilizers. On the other hand, a deficit of noradrenaline could also trigger emotional arousal. As with the serotonergic system, further research is needed before a definite link with Alzheimer's behaviors can be firmly established.

Somatostatin

Role in the brain and Alzheimer's disease

Among the other neurotransmitter chemicals suspected of playing a role in Alzheimer's are the neuropeptides: somatostatin, substance P, neurotensin, and cholecystokin (Perry and Perry

1985). Neuropeptides are peptides made from amino acids which are now known to function as neurotransmitters in the brain.

A lack of somatostatin also appears to contribute to Alzheimer's dementia. In particular, a lack of somatostatin appears to accompany the disease and contribute some to its impairments. Although research on this chemical is still in the early stages, somatostatin has been shown to be significantly reduced in several brain areas, including the parietal lobe, a region thought by many to be affected first and most profoundly in Alzheimer's disease (Tamminga et al. 1987). Other recent findings suggest that a loss of somatostatin neurons may be directly related to Alzheimer's dementia (Tamminga et al. 1987). While many questions remain about the role of somatostatin, the most current research suggests that it may be second only to acetylcholine in its importance for Alzheimer's disease.

Treating Neurotransmitter Deficiencies

Drug interventions Some drug treatments already exist for treating deficits in the cholinergic system, although to date they have not proven particularly effective. It may be that this system needs to be treated in conjunction with other affected systems. As research into the disease and its effects on the brain continue, it is highly likely that other neurotransmitters and chemical systems that have a bearing on Alzheimer's disease will be discovered as well. Because the disease's symptoms can vary widely from one individual to the next, it may be that a number of different neurochemical deficiencies are involved. A given individual's symptoms could hold the clue to treatment: a patient suffering from early dementia, pronounced visual-spatial deficits, and lesser intellectual and memory impairment, for example, might be more responsive to cholinergic drug treatment alone.

Other drug treatments for other chemical systems are likely to be discovered.

As we learn more about the full range of neuro-transmitter and other chemical deficiencies associated with Alzheimer's disease, it seems likely that drug treatments will become available which can at least partially compensate for these deficits and the problems they cause.

Summary

The levels of certain neurotransmitters and related chemicals crucial to the brain's information-communication process are lowered by Alzheimer's disease. The absence of these chemicals may cause the destruction of neurons, particularly the cholinergic neurons, that form the pathways to the hippocampus, the frontal/parietal lobes, and other areas of the brain's cortex. By cutting off effective communication between these areas, chemical disturbances in the brain may be responsible for many of the emotional, cognitive, memory, and behavioral changes suffered by Alzheimer's disease patients. Most Alzheimer's disease treatment-oriented research has sought ways to correct chemical abnormalities.

15

TREATMENT POSSIBILITIES

Role of drugs in Alzheimer's treatment
As medical researchers gradually come to understand the physical and chemical changes that occur in the Alzheimer's brain, they can use their knowledge to develop treatments that effectively prevent or reverse these changes. Many experimental studies using drug therapies on Alzheimer's patients already have been tried, with varying degrees of success. While no "wonder drug" for Alzheimer's disease—or even a clear and consistent treatment approach—has yet emerged, research has shown that some drugs help some of the people some of the time. Unfortunately, the studies completed thus far often show puzzling inconsistencies in response from one patient to the next. To achieve more consistent results, we no doubt need to learn more about the nature of the illness and its causes.

Cholinergic deficits target of treatment
To date, several major groups of drugs have been investigated. Many of the drug interactions in research have attempted to correct the deficiencies in the brain's cholinergic system. Since the neurotransmitter acetylcholine is deficient in the Alzheimer's brain and these deficiencies have been associated with Alzheimer's related impairments, it has been thought that finding ways to increase this chemical messenger might hold promise in treating the disease.

Basis for drug research

Additionally, lecithin and choline, which increase the availability of acetylcholine, have received some research attention. Drugs such as physostigmine and THA, which make acetylcholine available longer in the brain by blocking its destruction, have seemed promising in developing an effective treatment of Alzheimer's disease. Both drugs which directly increase the amount of acetylcholine and those that prevent its chemical destruction are called cholinergic agents.

In 1993, the Federal Drug Administraton (FDA) approved the use of THA under the name tacrine hydrochloride (Cognex). Recently a similar medication, donepezil (Aricept), was approved by the FDA. Both drugs are known as cholinesterase inhibitors because they slow the breakdown of the neurotransmitter, acetylcholine, and enhance its availabilty at the synapse so that information transmission is more likely to occur. These drugs depend upon a fairly intact system of neurons, their processes, and synaptic connectons. They will be more effective for persons with mild to moderate dementia.

As the result of epidemiologic research, two kinds of drugs that can prevent or slow the development of Alzheimer's disease have been identified—estrogen and anti-inflammatory agents. The use of another type of drugs, antioxidants, also promises to aid in the survival of neurons by the prevention or inhibition of oxidation. Free radicals generated through oxidative mechanisms are thought to play a role in Alzheimer's disease. A fine balance exists between oxygen free radical formation and antioxidant defense. When the balance is tipped in favor of the reactive free radical, oxidative stress results, thus making neurons especially vulnerable to free radical attack (Markesbery 1996). The accumulation of damage resulting from oxidation then causes nerve cells to degenerate.

In this chapter, we will look in turn at each of these groups of drugs and their effects. In addition, we will look at drug combination treatments and examine a nondrug therapy—neuronal transplants—that may hold a promise for the future. We also will discuss possible explanations for the inconsistent results of drug studies to date, including the possibility that Alzheimer's disease has distinct subtypes that respond to different treatments. First, however, we will discuss the issues that should be considered before one decides to participate in drug-research study.

Should You Participate in Drug-Research Study?

Participants in a drug-research study should carefully consider the risks and costs involved, as well as their own motivations.

In order for Alzheimer's treatments to be adequately developed and tested, it is necessary to conduct research using human subjects who have Alzheimer's disease. Subjects who volunteer for such studies do a great service both for medical research and for their fellow Alzheimer's sufferers. However, it is important that persons who elect to participate in a research study clearly understand the study's potential risks, results, and requirements, as well as their personal motivation for participating.

Families and subjects must not hold unrealistic expectations of significant improvement. Generally, persons with severe impairment have little chance of benefitting from drug treatment, while those in earlier stages of the disease may experience substantial, little, or no improvement. The drugs used might even cause a worsening of the patient's condition. Also, families and subjects sometimes cannot be told whether the subject will in fact be receiving the treatment medication or a placebo used for the control group.

Issues to consider

Other issues that must be carefully considered include:

- Purpose and rationale of study
- How study will be conducted
- Size and safety of dosage given
- Method of administering drug
- Potential side effects
- Responsibilities of the family
- Consent of the subject
- All expenses connected with participation (including travel, lodging, etc.)
- Researchers' attitude toward study participants (including family members)
- Researchers' credentials.

Inconsistencies in Drug Studies

Many unknown or uncontrolled variables may affect the results of studies, producing inconsistent findings.

Many uncontrolled variables exist in drug studies that may account for the frustrating inconsistencies found in Alzheimer's research. Among the many individual factors which may vary from one subject to the next, affecting or masking a drug's effects in a study include:

- Degree of subject's dementia
- Severity of loss of cholinergic neurons
- Incorrect diagnosis of Alzheimer's
- Coexisting disabilities (i.e., stroke)
- Other coexisting conditions (i.e., infection)
- Unrelated fluctuations in behavior and mood
- Age at onset of dementia.

Researchers do not yet know which variables may prove to be significant.

For example, a severe presenile dementia (onset before age 65) may be intrinsically different in terms of brain pathology than a severe senile dementia (onset after age 65), and thus it may respond very differently to a certain drug treatment. Any of the variables listed above may or may not prove to be an important indicator for Alzheimer's and drug research.

Other variables that must be controlled related to the study itself. These include:

- Dosage amounts
- Length of treatment and study
- Method of administration (òral, intravenous, etc.)
- Ways of measuring improvement
- Assumptions about the drug and effects expected
- Choice of symptoms to be measured.

Alzheimer's disease may prove to have distinct subtypes that respond differently to treatment.

Another possible explanation for the inconsistencies found is that Alzheimer's disease may have distinct subtypes, each associated with slightly different manifestations of symptoms and rate of progression. Different subtypes may respond differently to the same drug treatment. One researcher posits that two subtypes of Alzheimer's disease exist: AD-1 and AD-2 (Bondareff 1983).

As defined, AD-1 begins in old age and follows a slow, subtle progression; AD-2 begins in middle age and shows a more rapid course and greater impairment. Other neurochemical and anatomical differences established between the two groups would seem to support this distinction. For example, AD-2 might develop under more genetically controlled influence.

Another researcher has suggested four distinct subtypes of the disease: extrapyramidal, myclonic, benign, and typical (Mayeux et al. 1985). As compared to the typical group, the extrapyramidal and myclonic groups each show certain accentuated features, while the benign group shows underexpressed features. The groups also differ as to severity of impairment in cognitive and memory functions.

Attention to subtypes may produce better treatment strategies.

Other researchers now are looking into the validity and significance of the subtypes, and overall, the concept of subtypes may prove rewarding to research treatments. It may be that attention to these subtypes, and to other distinguishing indicators such as age of onset and severity of dementia, will lead to the creation of better drug-treatment strategies with more predictable and reliable results.

Despite the many variables to be controlled and the inconsistencies found in studies to date, it has been shown definitively that drug therapies can produce improvements in Alzheimer's symptoms. The challenge now is to identify some clear pattern that will show us which drugs can be expected to help which patients, in what ways, and for how long.

Cholinergic Agents

As we saw in the Chapter 14 discussion of chemical changes, Alzheimer's disease is accompanied by a lowered level of the neurotransmitter acetylcholine in the brain. Insufficient acetylcholine causes dysfunction of the brain's cholinergic system, which may lead in turn to impairment of memory and cognitive abilities.

Cholinergic agents are drugs that increase the brain's level of acetylcholine. Among the first treatments for Alzheimer's to be explored, then, are drugs that can increase the level of acetylcholine in the brain. The drugs tried include two substances that are precursors of acetylcholine: choline and lecithin. These substances increase the availability of acetylcholine. We will consider also physostigmine and THA which prevent the breakdown of this neurotransmitter. In this role, these two drugs prolong the availability of the acetylcholine. Finally, we will consider drugs that make the receptors for acetylcholine more sensitive, essentially heightening the potency of the available acetylcholine.

Choline

Choline therapy has produced extremely modest improvements. A component of various foods and of commercially available lecithin, choline can increase the availability of acetylcholine in the brain and enhance its synthesis and release in synapses between the neurons. Because of these potential effects, it first was approached with a great deal of hope. In the numerous studies completed, however choline therapy has been associated only with extremely modest improvements in Alzheimer's patients or no improvements at all.

In some cases a modest increase in alertness and awareness has been reported, although the increase has been accompanied by mild irritability; in a few others, a reduction in confusion has been noted

(Fovall et al. 1983). But all of these improvements have been so mild that they could have been simply ordinary behavioral fluctuations unrelated to the choline therapy. Those patients who have appeared to improve were in the earlier stages of the illness; no effect from choline therapy seems possible in more advanced cases. Some research findings suggest that choline might prove more beneficial when used in combination with other drugs.

Side effects from choline include nausea, abdominal pain, diarrhea, incontinence, and fishy odor in the sweat. This last side effect has been avoided by substituting phosphatidylcholine, a more complex form of the drug of which choline is a component. The availability of choline and lecithin encourage their use.

Lecithin

Lecithin is a naturally occurring dietary substance found in many foods, including egg yolks, meat, fish, and soybean products. The dosages of lecithin used in treating Alzheimer's disease, however, are much higher than those obtainable through a healthy diet. Like choline, lecithin increases the availability of acetylcholine; it also raises the body's blood choline level and maintains that level longer than does straight choline (Etienne 1983). It has been shown to produce small improvements in some patients.

Lecithin appears to slow deterioration in some patients. The most important finding is that lecithin could be capable of slowing deterioration in a few patients. This may mean that long-term lecithin therapy can be used to slow down the disease's progress (Dysken 1987). Supporting this theory is the finding in the Dysken study that patients who discontinued use of lecithin showed more rapid deterioration. However, this very limited evidence must be replicated in other studies before stronger conclusions can be drawn.

Lecithin may be an effective supplement to other drug therapies. At present, lecithin treatment requires further exploration. No compelling evidence suggests that it alone can produce significant or consistent improvement, though it may prove an effective supplement to other drug therapies. (This will be discussed in a later section.) Furthermore, there is no scientific evidence in support of the idea that lecithin can prevent Alzheimer's. Lecithin therapy has shown some very modest improvements in some patients some of the time. The idea behind lecithin and choline, increasing the amount of acetylcholine, remains a promising direction for future research.

Side effects of lecithin can include nausea, diarrhea, irritability, and dry mouth. These are more likely to occur in older persons. Lecithin is not otherwise harmful. It can be purchased in health food stores, but that form is usually 20 percent lecithin (Henig 1981). It would be impossible to take enough of this form of lecithin to be of any benefit with Alzheimer's disease.

Physostigmine

How physostigmine works

This drug works by slowing down the chemical destruction of acetylcholine in the brain's synapses. By keeping the existing acetylcholine available longer, it increases cholinergic activity at active synapses, although it cannot help synapses that have been damaged or destroyed by the disease. Since physostigmine is thought to effectively cross the blood-brain barrier (Smith et al. 1979), it will be more effective in blocking the breakdown of acetylcholine by the enzyme, acetylcholinesterase.

Physostigmine has produced modest improvements in memory that are greater than the results with either choline or lecithin.

A danger of physostigmine is its narrow dose range: only a slight difference exists between a safe dose and one that is toxic. Additionally, it does not stay in the body very long; thus it must be given more frequently. Despite the disadvantages, more positive results have been achieved with physostigmine than with either choline or lecithin. The improvements noted are modest: in mid-sized dosed, it improves verbal recognition memory; in larger doses, it improves nonverbal recognition memory (Dysken 1987). Overall, it seems to have positive effects on visual memory, that is, memory of information that is presented in a visual form (e.g., recognizing pictures).

Physostigmine also seems to improve certain types of learning measured by psychological tests, and the improvement is the greatest in patients with only mild symptoms. It will not be as effective when other neurotransmitter systems are impaired in addition to the cholinergic system—a condition that seems to be more frequent with early onset dementia (Mohs et al. 1985).

Studies encouraging but variable Overall, the studies with physostigmine are encouraging. Because they have shown such widely varying kinds and degrees of improvement—including no improvement in many patients—further research is needed to pinpoint the best uses for this drug: the most effective doses, the types of functions improved by various doses, and the kinds of patients who respond best. It is now available to researchers in oral form. The potential for toxicity can be monitored although it remains a risk factor for physostigmine. Although this drug has not produced dramatic improvements and its effects on the progression of Alzheimer's disease have not been determined, physostigmine shows promise for further research.

Tacrine and Donepezil

Tacrine, or THA (Tetrahydroaminoacridine), as it was known in earlier studies, was the first drug to become available for usage outside of research settings. It received multicenter clinical trials, and in September 1993, it was approved by the U.S. Food and Drug Administration under the name tacrine (Cognex) for treatment of Alzheimer's disease, despite concerns about its effectiveness. It has the same chemical action as physostigmine; it slows the chemical breakdown of acetylcholine in the brain's synapses and allows the small amounts of neurotransmitter released to remain longer than usual at the synaptic junction. Presumably, this action would more effectively support the transmission of information at the synapse. Keeping the neurotransmitter at the synapse longer might make up for the deficiency that has already been identified in the cholinergic system of the Alzheimer's brain.

Tacrine has several advantages over physostigmine: (1) it is longer-acting (O'Conner 1986); (2) it has fewer side effects (Kaye et al. 1982; Sitaram et al. 1983); and (3) it also effectively crosses the blood-brain barrier (O'Conner 1986). The fact that it can be taken orally (instead of by injection) and has few known side effects gives it a distinct advantage for use in the elderly population who are most frequently the target of Alzheimer's.

Study of tacrine began in 1981. In that study 75 percent of the subjects showed subjectively measured improvement from treatment with tacrine alone (Summers et al. 1981). Another study by Summers in 1986 also indicated improvement (Summers et al. 1986). Studies reported by others have investigated tacrine with and without lecithin; lecithin is not essential and does not contribute much to the therapeutic effect (Stern and Davis 1996). The effect of tacrine is described as being equivalent to slowing cognitive deterioration by 6 to 12 months. Such a length of time without further deterioration in function can be meaningful to patients and their caregivers.

The patient response to tacrine has been varied. Large benefits were experienced by 10 percent of patients. More modest benefits were demonstrated by 20 percent, and 20 percent showed smaller but significant improvement in clinical status or performance. Remaining patients exhibited no short-term benefits (Stern and Davis 1996).

Tacrine can be prescribed by one's family physician or another specialist, such as a psychiatrist or a neurologist. Adverse effects like nausea, belching, and diarrhea might occur, and blood tests will be needed to monitor liver function. Rash, anorexia, and rhinitis are other fairly common adverse effects.

The newer cholinesterase inhibitor, donepezil (Aricept), is more selective for the cholinesterase in the central nervous system; it will have fewer of the peripheral cholinergic effects like nausea, vomiting, and diarrhea. Liver function tests will not be necessary. It is indicated for persons with mild to moderate dementia of the Alzheimer's type. Dosage will be easy, since 5 mg. or 10 mg. can be given at bedtime. Adverse effects reportedly are mild and transient and are resolved during treatment with the medication.

The brain deficit of the neurotransmitter acetylcholine is probably only one of a cascade of biochemical events occurring in Alzheimer's disease. Since it is not likely to be the central event of the disease, treatments based solely on reversing the cholinergic deficiency could not be expected to be completely successful. Potential treatments for Alzheimer's disease have been expanded significantly for this reason.

Cholinergic Receptor Agonists

Studies of cholinergic receptor agonists have not produced significant improvements.

Other drugs that seem to help the brain's cholinergic system are cholinergic receptor agonists. These drugs work by stimulating the receptors that receive acetylcholine. Two such drugs, arecoline and RS-86, have been tried in studies on Alzheimer's patients, but unfortunately they produced little or no significant improvement (Bruno et al. 1986). Another drug, bethanacol chloride, did produce improvements such as decreased confusion, increased initiative, and greater productive activity in a four-subject study (Dysken 1987).

Administering drugs with a drug pump may allow more accurate research findings.

One interesting aspect of the bethanacol study was the pioneering drug-administration technique used. A drug infusing pump was implanted into the subject's abdominal wall and connected to an intracranial catheter (Dysken 1987). The pump allowed the drug to reach the brain directly and to cross the blood-brain barrier; it also allowed direct measurement of the amount of drug in the brain, something impossible with other administration techniques. The pump's improved measurement abilities, together with the steady, guaranteed dosage it provides, may make it a more desirable administration technique for all studies of brain-altering chemicals, allowing more precise findings. These benefits, however, must be weighed against the undesirable physical intrusiveness of the pump and catheter.

Naloxone and Naltrexone

Naloxone and Naltrexone have not been shown effective against Alzheimer's. Treatment with these drugs represents a very sophisticated investigation of the role of more fundamental biological systems of the brain affected by dementing illnesses. Although they have been tried on Alzheimer's patients in several studies, they have failed to produce any real, consistent improvement. Only one study with Naloxone has shown significant benefits from the drug (Reisberg, Ferris, et al. 1983). Several others have found the drug to exacerbate undesirable symptoms. At present, there is little evidence to suggest that these drugs hold promise for future treatment.

Vasodilators and Nootropic Agents

Vasodilators improve blood flow to the brain. Vasodilators are a group of drugs that improves blood flow to the brain by expanding narrowed blood vessels. In a brain stricken by Alzheimer's disease, a rapid and diffuse reduction in cerebral blood flow occurs after the onset of symptoms; vasodilators can help offset this reduction. In fact, vasodilators are more effective in raising cerebral blood flow in Alzheimer's patients than in normal persons of the same age (Reisberg 1981) or in persons with arteriosclerotic brain changes often referred to as "hardening of the arteries."

Two types of vasodilators exist: primary and secondary. Primary vasodilators—such as Nylidrin, the only one drug shown to improve dementia—act directly on vascular deficiencies. Secondary vasodilators—such as hydergine and piracetam, discussed next—increase blood flow indirectly by stimulating cerebral metabolism. Metabolism is a chemical process necessary for the body and brain to maintain and regenerate themselves. Energy is a product of metabolism.

Cerebral blood flow has a strong relationship with metabolic activity. Disturbances in metabolism seem tied to reductions in cerebral blood flow found in Alzheimer's disease. For instance, persons with

Alzheimer's have significantly lower levels of oxygen and glucose utilization in the frontal, temporal, and parietal areas of the brain. Secondary vasodilators stimulate the brain's metabolism to increase cerebral blood flow. The following secondary vasodilators show some promise for treating Alzheimer's disease.

Piracetam

Another cerebral metabolic enhancer, piracetum is also one of the nootropic agents—a group of compounds that seems to improve functioning in mild to moderate senile dementia (Jenike 1985). Piracetam increases the response of neurons in the hippocampus (Cooper 1984) and appears to stimulate cerebral glucose metabolism (Jenike et al. 1986) and enhance release of acetylcholine in the hippocampus (Rosenberg et al. 1983).

Piracetam may improve memory and learning. In animal studies, piracetam has increased brain energy reserves, increased learning, and protected against learning impairment. The same studies indicate that piracetam does not have side effects or toxic effects at normal therapeutic doses (Schneck 1983). Preliminary evidence suggests that a combination of piracetam and choline given for one week improved memory storage, recall, and delayed recall (Schneck 1983). It may be that piracetam is most effective when combined with drugs that increase the availability of acetylcholine. As with other drug treatments, more mildly impaired patients—those whose cholinergic systems are least damaged and thus most responsive—seem to show the greatest benefit. This drug needs more research studies to determine whether it can be useful in treatment of Alzheimer's disease.

Neuropeptides

Neuropeptides are short chains of amino acids that have strong effects on the nervous system. Certain types of neuropeptides act as hormones in the body and have roles as neurotransmitters in the brain; they also assist in the communication between body cells, tissues, and organs (Reisberg 1981). Research into possible uses for neuropeptides in treating Alzheimer's is still in the early stages.

Neuropeptides may improve memory, learning, and mood, and hold promise as general geriatric antidepressants.

In animal studies, neuropeptides have produced reversal of memory impairment. They also have been shown to boost human cognitive abilities, to play a role in neurotransmission, and in memory and learning. However, drug research with Alzheimer's patients to date has not been particularly encouraging results. Neuropeptides have been shown to produce mood improvements such as reduced depression, increased energy, and increased attention and concentration (Ferris 1983), and they may prove to have a role as geriatric antidepressants.

Vasopressin

Both a neuropeptide and a secondary vasodilator, vasopressin has improved memory and learning in animal studies. In one particularly interesting study with rats, vasopressin helped the animals remember things they had previously forgotten. In a study with Alzheimer's patients who suffered memory disturbances, use of a vasopressin nasal spray helped memories appear more quickly. Normal adult men have shown improved attention, concentration, and recall in response to vasopressin (Reisberg 1982).

Vasopressin and its analogs may improve memory, concentration, and mood.

Vasopressin analogs—such as LVP, ODAVP, and DGAVP—also have been tried on Alzheimer's patients, with mixed results. One study has shown small but statistically significant improvements in memory, retrieval, and reaction time when an analog was administered (Ferris 1983). Possibly the more potent, longer-acting analogs will prove to have the greatest effects. Further research is needed to determine how vasopressin and its analogs work: by genuinely improving memory, by stimulating enhanced concentration, or by acting as an antidepressant.

Because of the role they seem to play in memory, learning, and communications between neurons, neuropeptides represent a promising frontier for further research. At the very least, they may prove helpful as antidepressant agents.

Psychostimulants

This group of drugs stimulated the central nervous system, increasing motor activity and reducing fatigue. Although psychostimulants do not improve cognitive or memory abilities, they can benefit other symptoms of Alzheimer's disease. Research has focused on treating three clusters of symptoms: (1) apathetic and withdrawn behavior, (2) mild depression, and (3) impaired short-term memory (Prien 1983).

Psychostimulants may improve attitude and mood. Of the psychostimulants tried, a number of drugs, such as ritalin, have generally proven unhelpful. These drugs may exacerbate behavior that is already agitated. Metrazol has received mixed reviews, but it has seemed to help with apathy, withdrawal, drive, and self-care (Prien 1983). However, it has a number of very undesirable side effects. Procaine hydrocholoride, the primary active ingredient in a drug called Gerovital-H3, seems to have potential only for the treatment of geriatric depression (Prien 1983).

To date, then, psychostimulants have not proven particularly helpful, although they may have some use in treating specific sub-types of Alzheimer's. The side effects associated with these drugs require that they be carefully monitored, however, and may limit their usefulness.

Combination Drug Studies

Lecithin and THA seem to work well together, complementing each other's action. Often two or more drugs are given in combination so that each can help the other do its job. As we saw in the 1986 Summers study, for example, THA and lecithin were successfully combined to produce different but complementary actions. The lecithin increased the availability of acetylcholine in the synapses between neurons, while the THA inhibited the activity of the enzyme that breaks acetylcholine down in the receiving neuron. Together they produced the desired effect: more usable acetylcholine in the brain. In another study, lecithin and THA were given together to a group of Alzheimer's subjects with relatively high education and an average of 61.5 years; some improvement in learning was noted, particularly among the more mildly impaired (Sitaram et al. 1983).

Lecithin has also been combined with choline and physostigmine. Lecithin has also been paired in studies with psysostigmine. One study noted some improvements in long-term memory when lecithin and physostigmine were given together (Peters and Levin 1982). Another study of the same drug pairing produced even more impressive results. Eight out of the 12 subjects showed clear improvements in recall from long-term memory and a decrease in intrusions—memories seemingly forgotten but later interjected into another context (Thal and Fuld .1983). The results were repeated in a subsequent trial. Somewhat surprisingly, other studies of this drug combination have shown a greater degree of improvement in more severely impaired subjects.

Combination drug treatments, like single drug treatments, generally have not shown the kind of consistent results for which one might hope. Subjects who share similar characteristics—such as degree of dementia, early or late onset of dementia (before or after age 65), and so fourth—do not seem to respond similarly to the drugs. This makes it very difficult to predict subject response or identify any pattern in the study results.

Estrogen, Anti-Inflammatory Agents, and Antioxidants

One way to think about slowing down or halting the destruction of Alzheimer's disease is to discover ways to protect and preserve the neurons of the brain and their synapses. Several disease-related processes conceivably produce cell death. Estrogen is a hormone that is thought to have important roles in the brain and other parts of the body in addition to its role in the female reproductive system. Like the antioxidants and anti-inflammatory drugs, estrogen may help nerve cells survive by preventing damage from inflammation and oxidation. There is growing evidence that estrogens serve a normal maintenance role in the same area of the brain most affected by Alzheimer's (Simpkins et al. 1994). Estrogen appears to promote the growth of cholinergic neurons and may interact with apolipoprotein E—factors that could affect the risk for Alzheimer's (Tang et al. 1996). Acting as a neurotropic factor, estrogen stimulates neurite growth and synapse formation in responsive neurons (Henderson et al. 1994). It also seems to work as an antioxidant by stopping the harmful action of oxygen molecules on cells and is thought to promote cell metabolism.

One study suggests that the increased incidence of Alzheimer's in older women may be due to estrogen deficiency. Estrogen replacement therapy may be useful for preventing or delaying the onset of Alzheimer's disease (Paganini-Hill and Henderson 1994). Earlier studies showed that women who had taken estrogen after menopause had lower rates of Alzheimer's than those who had not. Estrogen use has even been associated with better cognitive performance in women with Alzheimer's compared to others with the disease who did not use it (Henderson et al. 1994).

A significant role for estrogen may develop in Alzheimer's treatment or prevention. However, estrogen replacement therapy following menopause is not recommended for all women. This factor, and also the issue of how men might benefit from the protective role of estrogen, are some of the issues that need further investigation. Cholinergic neurons of the brain have numerous estrogen receptors, which occur on the same neurons that have receptors for nerve growth factor. Does this mean that estrogen and nerve growth factor have a common role in preventing the degeneration of cholinergic neurons? This is still being addressed by research.

Preventing damage associated with brain inflammation and oxidation helps nerve cells in the brain survive. Studies have shown that people who take anti-inflammatory drugs or suffer from inflammatory diseases like rheumatoid arthritis have a reduced risk of developing Alzheimer's disease. Another study shows that there is a low incidence of Alzheimer's in Japanese leprosy patients who have continuously taken a medication that has anti-inflammatory activity. One study indentifying the protective role of anti-inflammatories notes that the role may be greater in people over 70. Anti-inflammatory treatment was more effective in those without the apoE4 allele (Breitner 1996). Anti-inflammatory agents include steroidal ones like prednisone and non-steroidal anti-inflammatory drugs labeled NSAIDS, including such over-the-counter drugs as aspirin and ibuprofen. Indomethacin and naproxen are examples that require a prescription.

A recently released study indicates that those taking NSAIDS had half the risk of developing the disease that the people who did not use the drugs. The researchers also established for the first time that longer use of these drugs decreases the risk of Alzheimer's disease. Shorter-term use might also reduce the risk. The most commonly used anti-inflammatory drug was ibuprofen. Aspirin and acetaminophen, which is not an NSAID, had little or no effect on reducing risk, though the aspirin dosages may have been too low to affect the central nervous system (Stewart et al. 1997).

A 6-month study of indomethacin showed that Alzheimer's patients who took the NSAID had stable cognition. Function declined in those patients who had not taken the drug. Adverse effects must be carefully monitored and might limit its use in some persons (Aisen and Davis 1994).

The reader is reminded that these findings are still preliminary, and potentially serious adverse effects are assoicated with the chronic use of anti-inflammatory drugs—for instance, gastric irritation and bleeding, peptic ulcer disease, and even impaired kidney function. Any ongoing use should be supervised by a physician.

Aging and Alzheimer's disease are assoicated with increased free radical formation. Oxidative stress results when antioxidant defenses are overwhelmed by free radical formation. Free radicals can also be caused by the beta amyloid protein, glutamate, or other toxic factors. Antioxidants protect neurons from oxidative damage and could have beneficial effects in Alzheimer's by reducing the free radical formation and preventing the associated cell injury and loss.

Selegiline, or deprenyl, is used in the treatment of Parkinson's disease. It is also an antioxidant. Selegiline and vitamin E (alphtocopherol) are both presumed to reduce oxidative stress and believed to have neuroprotective functions. Vitamin E traps free radicals and interrupts the chain reaction that damages cells. It also prevents cell death caused by glutamate and beta amyloid protein. Selegiline is thought to act as a scavenger of free radicals (Shihabuddin and Davis 1996). It may improve cognitive deficits.

The results of a long-anticipated study involving selegiline and vitamin E, given separately and in combination to patients with Alzheimer's, have recently been published (Sano et al. 1997). The authors focused on functional losses instead of cognitive deterioration. Both drugs were reported to delay functional deterioration. There were no differences reported between the results of the group receiving the combined treatment and either of the groups receiving individual treatments. Falls and transient loss of consciousness were noted to be more frequent in treatment groups. Treatment with selegiline and vitamin E slows the progession of the disease in patients with moderately severe Alzheimer's disease, and is recommended for persons with moderate dementia.

Such findings will always face serious questions. More study of these drugs must be carried out to determine their value in long-term management of Alzheimer's. Both drugs are available: vitamin E is available everywhere over the counter, and a prescription is needed for selegiline. Those caring for persons with this disease may wish to try one or the other of the drugs with the guidance of their physician.

Neuronal Transplants

In the future, it may become possible to transplant healthy neurons to certain brain areas and thus regenerate brain function.

In the future, it may be possible to graft healthy neuronal tissue onto impaired areas of the Alzheimer's brain, thus stimulating the regeneration of neuron networks and improving certain brain functions. This transplant technique could offer an important alternative for more severly impaired victims, since drug therapies rarely seem to help those with extensive neuron damage.

Neuronal transplants already have been tried on subjects suffering from Parkinson's disease. One such study reported a slowing of degeneration (Moore 1987), while another reported an improvement in motor functioning (Madrazo et al. 1987). Animal research with neuronal transplants has shown that the technique can achieve desired results for specific behavioral and cognitive impairments (Gash et al. 1985; Merz 1987; Fine 1986; Gage et al. 1984).

Finding sources for donor tissue raises delicate ethical questions.

Before neuronal transplants can be widely used, however, the sensitive issue of donor tissue must be resolved. In the latest Parkinson's disease study, dopamine-producing cells were simply transplanted from the patient's own adrenal glands. An equivalent source of acetylcholine-producing cells from the patient's own body for treating Alzheimer's disease is not yet known if it does exist. It may be possible to use fetal brain tissue from some other animal; an even better source of donor tissue would be the brains of aborted human fetuses. Animal studies with grafted fetal tissue have been quite successful, although the technique has not been tested with human neuronal tissue. The use of either animal or fetal tissue, however, raises serious moral and ethical questions that would first have to be addressed.

Most likely, years of animal research will need to be completed before experimentation with human subjects can even be considered. Perhaps in that time, the ethical questions surrounding this treatment possibility will be answered as well. Neuronal transplants are an experimental possiblility for research at this time.

Nerve growth factors

Nerve cells outside the body's central nervous system have the caspacity to be regenerated after being damaged. The nerve cells of the brain do not seem to have this ability. These cells and others in the body do develop in specific patterns under the direction of special chemicals called "nerve growth factors." Scientists are now investigating these chemicals to determine if they might be used to regrow or regenerate deteriorating nerve cells in the brain (Mace and Rabins 1991). If this process were better understood it might be possible to stimulate the replacement or regrowth of damaged brain cells. This, in turn, could allow treatment with medications to be better utilized. Some restoration of the pathway necessary for the brain's chemical messengers might be possible.

16

PSYCHIATRIC MEDICATIONS AND DEMENTIA

Psychiatric medications can be effective in managing some symptoms of Alzheimer's.

Psychiatric medications can be effective in managing some symptoms of Alzheimer's disease. An overview of these various medications will be helpful to caregivers. Since side effects, some quite adverse, can develop, these medications require close monitoring by physicians and family members. Individual responses to psychiatric medications can vary considerably, from clear benefits, to no change, to even worse symptoms. The elderly generally have a lower tolerance for these medications than younger persons, and brain impairments often interfere with the effectiveness of a medication.

A good rule of thumb with psychiatric medications is to start persons at low dosages, increasing dosages slowly. This approach may be frustrating to family members who are seeking rapid relief from some symptoms. It is a safer approach, however, and allows physicians to monitor an individual's response to a medication. Side effects are more likely to occur at higher dosages. If the person is going to experience adverse side effects, these probably will occur in a milder form at a lower dose. Additionally, it is critical to determine over a period of time whether a person can tolerate a specific psychiatric medication; lower doses allow the body to gradually adjust to the medication.

No one but a physician should change prescribed dosages.

Only physicians should change dosages. Family members should consult the physician if side effects develop or if the medication is simply not working. Families should have realistic expectations about changes they can expect; generally medications can produce moderate changes. Target symptoms should be discussed with the prescribing physician, who must be informed of any other medications the patient is currently taking. Family must not change the dosage even if behaviors such as agitation or angry outbursts are still occurring. In fact, more of the medication could create more severe symptoms, which is especially true with major tranquilizers. Administering more medication than prescribed can also create more side effects, which can be dangerous, especially for the person with Alzheimer's disease. The following example illustrates some problems associated with increasing the dosage of a major tranquilizer without the advice of a physician.

A case example illustrating the harmful effect of too high a dosage of a major tranquilizer

Emma Day, an elderly woman, had been prescribed a 150 mg total daily dosage of a major tranquilizer. This particular medication (Mellaril) had high sedative effects. The dosage had been increased over a month to reduce symptoms of agitation, sleeping difficulties, and delusional beliefs about her husband. These symptoms were reduced but still occurred occasionally. Jim, the husband, had diabetes and severe arthritis. The diabetes was not well-controlled, thus causing periods of depression.

On this particular day, Jim was somewhat agitated himself due to fatigue and worry over caregiving and financial problems. He was abrupt and aggravated with Emma's slowness in bathing. He saw her behavior as resistant and uncooperative. As he became more forceful, Emma became more upset. The more he pushed, the more hostile she became. Later she calmed down, but Jim decided on his own to increase her medication. That night he doubled the dosage.

The next morning Emma was a little more confused and sedated; Jim doubled the dosage again. Later that morning she was still in bed, and Jim wanted her to get up. He got her out of bed with some difficulty, pointed her toward the bathroom, and left for another part of the house. On his way he heard her fall. She was not seriously injured, but her shoulder and elbow were badly bruised. For several weeks, Jim had to help her more with dressing and bathing. Emma's fall and Jim's increased workload were direct results of too much tranquilizer given without a doctor's order.

Major tranquilizers generally should not be used as chemical restraint. Except in extraordinary circumstances the use of major tranquilizers as a chemical restraint is inappropriate. This should never be done at home by family members. Two other points are made in the example above: (1) caregivers, particularly those who are older, often have health problems that can interfere with caregiving and their response to daily stressors, and (2) it is to the benefit of the caregiver and patient to use problem-solving and coping skills, rather than to increase medication.

In this chapter, we will cover three groups of medications used in treating symptoms associated with dementia or other coexisting psychiatric conditions, such as depression. Side effects will be discussed and listed by groups of medications that may produce them. The reasons these medications are prescribed, as well as their generic and brand names, will be noted.

Side Effects

Major tranquilizers are the most frequently prescribed medications for symptoms associated with dementia. One potential side effect that must be monitored is *hypotension*. This results in a lowering of blood pressure, which can increase the risk of falls caused by dizziness and loss of balance.

Another type of side effect is called *extrapyramidal reactions,* which causes decreased or slowed movements, muscle rigidity, resting hand tremor, shuffling gait, drooling, and a mask-like face. Some of these symptoms can accompany dementia particularly if true Parkinson's disease coexists with Alzheimer's disease. The drug-induced or "pseudoparkinsonism" is likely to appear sometime between the first week and two months after beginning treatment with a major tranquilizer. These symptoms can be reduced with careful additions of other medications, which in turn may be discontinued later if the symptoms fade.

When major tranquilizers are given to reduce agitation and restlessness but instead produce these symptoms, the person is having a "paradoxical reaction" to the medication. The patient cannot sit still, may be constantly pacing, and feels anxious and agitated. In addition, the person may find it difficult to sleep; no position is comfortable. A change in medication, reducing the dosage, or use of an antiparkinson-type medication might help some people with this side effect.

If persons with Alzheimer's disease have taken major tranquilizers for a long time, they run the risk of another type of extrapyramidal reaction called "tardive dyskinesia." Advancing age can also be a risk factor. This type of side effect is characterized by involuntary lip and tongue motions and writhing movements of the arms and legs. In more severe tardive dyskinesia speech, eating, walking, and even breathing can be impaired. Reducing the dosage or adding an antiparkinson medication does not consistently help reduce this side effect. The best treatment is preventive; that is, avoid the use of major tranquilizers whenever possible or use low dosages.

Another possible side effect is a delirium or reversible dementia that is related to an anticholinergic effect some major tranquilizers can have. The more common features involve dry mouth, blurred vision, dilated pupils, constipation, urinary retention, nasal congestion, and increased heart rate. A few major tranquilizers can inhibit ejaculation. The cholinergic system of the brain, which is vital to memory functions, is already impaired in Alzheimer's disease. Major tranquilizers and some classes of antidepressants block the function of acetylcholine, the chemical messenger intrinsic to the cholinergic neurons of the brain.

In addition, a syndrome can develop which appears as an acute, toxic confusional state. This state is characterized by disorientation, visual hallucinations, irritability, and impaired attention. The syndrome can be treated by discontinuing the drug(s) with anticholinergic effects. Symptoms should clear in two to three days. The medication can then be changed to one with less anticholinergic properties or resumed if the syndrome developed from a toxic buildup.

Several other side effects can occur with some major tranquilizers. One which applies particularly to elderly persons is greater sensitivity to heat and cold. Weight gain can also occur when taking major tranquilizers. Cardiac side effects, while rare with some of the major tranquilizers, are possible and must be taken into consideration for those patients with heart conditions.

Other side effects can occur but are quite rare. Family members should consult a physician when the Alzheimer's patient is prescribed any type of medication in order to monitor side effects.

Three groups of psychiatric medications, major tranquilizers, minor tranquilizers, and antidepressants, are described in the tables that follow.

Major Tranquilizers
(Neuroleptics or Antipsychotics)

Purpose: Manage symptoms of agitation/anxiety, suspiciousness, hostility, delusions, hallucinations, preoccupations, poor self-care resulting from psychotic state, social withdrawal, uncooperativeness, belligerent and hostile behavior.

Drugs have a tranquilizing or sedating effect. There is an antipsychotic effect or normalizing effect on mood, thought, and behavior.

Side Effects:

Drowsiness	Sensitivity to light	Decreased sweating
Dry mouth	Shakiness	Difficulty urinating
Constipation	Muscle spasms in neck/back	Restlessness
Blurred vision	Dizziness/light-headedness	Hypotension
Stiffness	Stuffy nose	Fast heartbeat
Drooling	Decreased sexual ability	Shuffling gait

Any side effects of concern should be brought to the attention of the physician prescribing the medication. The following table notes some common major tranquilizers and side effects.

MAJOR TRANQUILIZERS

Trade Name	Generic Name	Sedative	Anticholinergic	Extrapyramidal
High Potency				
Haldol	Haloperidol	Low	Low	High
Navane	Thiothixene	Low	Low	High
Prolixin	Fluphenazine			
	HCL	Low	Low	High
Stelazine	Trifluoperazine			
	HCL	Moderate	Low	Moderate
Moderate Potency				
Trilafon	Perphenazine	Moderate	Moderate	Moderate
Loxitane	Loxapine			
	Succinate	Moderate	Moderate	Moderate
Moban	Molindone HCL	Moderate	Moderate	Moderate
Low Potency				
Thorazine	Chlorpromazine	High	High	Low
Mellaril	Thioridazine	High	High	Low

Newer neuroleptic medications like risperidone (Risperdal) may be useful in the treatment of psychiatric symptoms associated with Alzheimer's disease due to their desired action and side effect profile. More specifics concerning their effectiveness will be known as more treatment history develops.

Minor Tranquilizers

Minor tranquilizers are used to treat some symptoms that accompany Alzheimer's disease. They may be more appropriate for controlling anxiety/agitation when psychotic features are not evident. These medications can build up in the body over time, thus those medications with shorter half-life should be used to prevent this buildup. The longer the half-life of a medication, the longer it stays in the body. We will note the half-live below and each drug's action rate (rate of onset). In some cases, it may be more appropriate to dispense this medication as needed rather than regularly. We will only note the antianxiety agents.

Purpose: Reduce symptoms of anxiety/agitation and related insomnia.

MINOR TRANQUILIZERS

Generic Name	Brand Name	Rate of Onset	Half-Life (Hours)	Dose Range mg/day for Elderly
Diazepam	Valium	Fastest	26–53	2–10
Clorazepate dipotassium	Tranxene	Fast	30–200	7.5–15
Triazolam	Halcion	Fast	2–5	.25–.5
Lorazepam	Ativan	Intermediate	20–200	.5–4
Chordiazepoxide HCl	Librium	Intermediate	8–28	5–30
Alprazolam	Xanax	Intermediate	6–15	.125–.5
Oxazepam	Serax	Intermediate to slow	5–15	10–30
Temazepam	Restoril	Intermediate to slow	12–24	15–30
Prazepam	Centrax	Slow	30–300	10–15

Side Effects:

Oversedation	Dizziness	Fatigue
Drowsiness	Light-headedness	Depression
Unusual excitement	Headache	Blurred vision
Nervousness	Irritability (paradoxical)	Breathing problems

As with other medications, use of minor tranquilizers may not be appropriate with other medical conditions. The physician will consider this factor. Withdrawal from this type medication should be supervised by a physician since there can be problems if the person has taken the medication for a long time.

Antidepressants

While there is some question about how often Alzheimer's patients are depressed, there is no question that depression can precede or coexist with Alzheimer's disease. Some depression (coexisting with Alzheimer's disease) can be treated successfully, and the person's mental status will improve. However, side effects are a major concern with antidepressants. Anticholinergic effects can occur with anti-

ANTIDEPRESSANTS

Generic Name	Brand Name	Sedation	Anticholinergic	Orthostatic Hypotension
Amitriptyline	Elavil	High	High	High
Amoxapine	Asendin	Moderate	Low	Moderate
Bupropion	Wellbutrin	Low	Low	Low
Clomipramine	Anafranil	High	High	High
Desipramine	Norpramin	Low	Low	Low
Doxepin	Sinnequan/Adapin	High	Moderate-High	High
Fluoxetine	Prozac	Low	Low	Low
Imipramine	Tofranil	Moderate	Moderate	Moderate
Maprotiline	Ludiomil	High	Low	Low
Nortriptyline	Pamelor/Aventyl	Low	Low	Low
Paroxetine	Paxil	Low	Low	Low
Sertraline	Zoloft	Low	Low	Low
Trazodone	Desyrel	High	Low	Moderate

depressant medications. While all side effects can be significant, those that produce more confusion and delirium must be prevented. In dementia, these effects compound existing memory and cognitive deficits. Careful use of the appropriate antidepressants can sometimes avoid these side effects. (See Chapter 3 for more detailed information about depression with Alzheimer's.)

Purpose: Decrease aspects of depressed mood, improve appetite and sleeping habits, improve social functioning, increased level of energy.

Side Effects:

Drowsiness	Increase in heart rate	Hypotension
Dry mouth	Blurred Vision	Arrythmias
Urinary retention	Constipation	Weight gain
Nasal congestion	Dizziness/fainting	Stomach upset
Delirium	Tremors	Nausea
Increased appetite for sweets	Slow pulse	

There is some interest in another type of antidepressant medication, the monamine oxidase inhibitors (MAOs or MAOIs). This antidepressant may be considered when others do not work. However, special care must be taken regarding dietary restrictions and combining with other medications. This type of medication also has side effects which must be carefully considered. Newer antidepressant medications known as Serotonin Selective Reuptake Inhibitors (SSRIs), which include sertraline and fluoxetine, tend to have desirable side effect profiles, especially for older individuals. For example, medications with strong indications of anticholinergic side effects and orthostatic hypotension (sudden drop in blood pressure when standing) are more likely to contribute to mental confusion and are a greater risk for falls.

Most antidepressant medications take several weeks to a month to reach a therapeutic level. Families must take this into account and be patient. With the elderly, a lower dosage is often indicated to determine how well the antidepressant will be tolerated.

Summary

Psychiatric medications—when carefully prescribed and monitored—can be helpful in the management of psychiatric symptoms assoicated with Alzheimer's disease. Family must understand why these medications are prescribed and what side effects can be expected. Many times a simple explanation will encourage Alzheimer's patients to take their medications. All psychiatric medications can help with "nerves," relaxation, and sleep. Families must be responsible for monitoring side effects and reporting these to the prescribing physician. Family members must avoid the temptation to exaggerate or overreport disturbing symptoms in order to increase prescribed dosages. Finally, the help of a professional should be sought to learn more appropriate ways to handle behavior problems and caregiver stress. Depending solely on psychiatric medications will not be sufficient.

AN AFTERWORD

When I was about 17, I found an old German drinking mug hidden among the rubble heaped along a creek near my grandparents' home in an isolated rural area near Waco, Texas. The creek, one of my favorite places, was exciting to explore, partly because I could hide in the sea cane and splash through the water, but also because I always hoped I would find something ancient and valuable there. My eyes alert for old coins and arrowheads, I would find instead rusty cans and buckles from old mule harnesses—until the day I spotted the old mug. The handle was broken, but as with many decorative mugs of its type, there were inscriptions on it in old German. Surely, I thought, there was some great truth revealed there, if only I could find someone to translate it.

My family had long since stopped speaking German and had largely forgotten the language, but I searched for someone to help me understand what the words meant. Finally, a high school German teacher found someone to translate the ancient German saying:

> God protect you.
> Things have happened
> Differently than I imagined

and

> God protect you.
> It would have been nice.

In my adolescent frame of mind, I thought at the time the inscription must have related to a long-ago youth who had lost his first love. Later when I began working with the elderly and their families, however, that saying deepened in meaning with an application to losses of a very different nature. It is hard to accept lost dreams, unfulfilled at the end of a brief romance. It is quite another thing to see plans and dreams made over decades slowly but unrelentingly ripped apart by an illness that seems to go on forever before it ends.

The ancient saying takes on new meaning when I look at it today, applying those words to the people I work with daily—victims of Alzheimer's and their families, engaged in a long good-bye filled with the acceptance of something that is not over, at least not yet.

I remember how the mug had been chipped in a number of places, the porcelain finish cracked from the ravages of time and weather. As a teenager, I imagined how beautiful the mug must have been long ago. I thought of all the history it could have shared with me if it could have talked. Many times, I tried to find ways to restore the mug to its original condition. The chips were filled in, but that did not help much. It was still chipped and could not be restored.

Finally, I accepted the mug for what it was. It was still special, and the message it carried became more meaningful as time passed. I could not put the mug back into its original shape. Its personal value to me cannot be fully appreciated by others. Its original function and purpose has been lost, but it still occupies an honorable place on a bookshelf in my home, and its message serves to remind me that life is full of losses and disappointments, but it is also full of hopes.

It is common to look back on what has happened, the good and the bad, when we have lost someone. In the case of Alzheimer's, your caregiving made a difference to the one you loved. You need to hear that now, to accept it, and to let it make a difference to you.

Any one of us could say that things have worked out differently than we imagined. If we are thinking of only what could have been, we are probably pondering how nice it could have been. We might ponder instead what was and still is—the experiences, the memories, and the accomplishments of one's whole life. And they are nice, too, aren't they?

Behut dich Gott,
(God Protect You)

Howard Gruetzner
Waco, Texas

APPENDIX A
WORKSHEETS

Use of the Behavior Profile

The "Behavior Profile" can be helpful to the family caregiver and professional. We will briefly discuss its contents and uses.

Behavioral areas: There are 58 behaviors listed in five categories. These behaviors occur with Alzheimer's disease although some may not occur as frequently in all persons. Certainly on an infrequent basis some occur with almost everyone. The difference is frequency. The behavior problem can occur with other conditions, particularly psychiatric disorders.

How often it occurs: Many problems are not significant unless they occur frequently. This is certainly the case with symptoms and their manifestations in Alzheimer's disease. More supervision may be indicated if a behavior occurs frequently, such as not eating or bathing; others need attention even if a behavior occurs infrequently, such as wandering or leaving the stove turned on. The caregiver can use the frequency of a behavior to plan the necessary degree of assistance and supervision. Some behaviors will require more intervention than others. Potential consequences of a behavior will influence the type of intervention and how quickly an intervention must be made. For instance, if a person begins to get lost driving, action must be taken to stop his driving. Denial of problems may occur. This will be bothersome but does not pose a problem unless the person insists on doing things anyway that could have harmful consequences.

How much it bothers you: This will help point out behaviors that need more understanding and attention. For instance, if toileting accidents are extremely bothersome to the caregiver, this area should be addressed to reduce the number of accidents. If the person has delusional ideas, these will probably be accompanied by agitation. These behaviors usually bother caregivers a great deal initially. Psychiatric medication will probably be needed. As caregivers are trying to adjust to the symptoms of Alzheimer's disease, they may be bothered more by a larger number of symptoms.

Completing the profile: For each behavior, check the most appropriate box under the two categories: *How often it occurs* and *How much it bothers you.* If the behavior is no longer a concern because you have taken over that area, scratch through the behavior and the row of boxes to the right. For example, if you pay bills for the person now, scratch through "forgets to pay bills" and the boxes to the right.

Use of the profile: Both caregivers and professionals can use the profile. Caregivers can complete the profile and refer to it to see how behaviors change and how their perception of problems change. The more seriously impaired person will have more behaviors occurring more frequently. This, however, usually occurs over time. If the frequency of numerous behaviors increases abruptly, an underlying medical condition may have developed. Medications might need to be reviewed.

If the person has not been diagnosed, the completed profile will provide information to the physician about the individual's functioning and the caregiver's concerns. The profile is not intended to be a diagnostic tool, but when a person is not testable, a reliable family informant can provide a more complete picture of functioning by completing the profile.

For counseling purposes the profile can indicate behaviors that need more problem-solving work and understanding. It also more quickly identifies behavior areas that are of great concern to the caregiver and thus require additional support and/or intervention.

BEHAVIOR PROFILE

NAME: _____ CAREGIVER: _____

DATE: _____ LENGTH OF CAREGIVING: _____

Check the appropriate category for each behavior.

BEHAVIORAL AREAS	How Often It Occurs				How Much It Bothers You				
	Always	Usually	Sometimes	Never	Extremely	Very much	Moderately	A little	Not at all
ORIENTATION									
1. Fails to recognize friends									
2. Fails to recognize family									
3. Forgets year									
4. Forgets month									
5. Forgets day of week									
6. Unable to name place (town, etc.)									
7. Fails to recognize familiar places									
8. Gets lost in neighborhood (walking)									
9. Gets lost driving									
10. Gets lost in own home									
11. More confused at night									
12. More confused in new places									
13. Wanders and gets lost									
MEMORY									
14. Loses/misplaces small items									
15. Loses/misplaces valuable things									
16. Forgets to pay bills									
17. Forgets to eat									
18. Unable to recall what was read									
19. Forgets to turn things off									
20. Forgets what conversation is about									
21. Unable to follow what's on TV									
22. Forgets to bathe									
23. Forgets major events of the day									
24. Forgets major events of the week									
25. Forgets major events from distant past									
LANGUAGE									
26. Unable to initiate conversation									
27. Misunderstands what others say									
28. Unable to respond to questions									
29. Has trouble finding right words									
30. Just speaks in phrases									
31. Avoids questions									

	How Often It Occurs				How Much It Bothers You				
	Always	Usually	Sometimes	Never	Extremely	Very much	Moderately	A little	Not at all
32. Unable to verbalize needs									
33. Repeatedly says same things									
34. What is said makes little sense									

AMBULATION/MOVEMENT

35. Walks short, shuffling gait									
36. Gait slow and labored									
37. Tires easily when walking									
38. Unable to get up from chair alone									
39. Unable to use stairs									
40. Unable to use eating utensils									
41. Unable to write name									
42. Hands/arms shake									

BEHAVIOR PROBLEMS

43. Has problems sleeping									
44. Has toileting accidents									
45. Talks excessively about past									
46. Denies problems									
47. Gets upset easily									
48. Becomes physically violent									
49. Shows poor judgment									
50. Has trouble taking medication									
51. Drives unsafely									
52. Very withdrawn, refuses to leave house									
53. Very nervous and restless									
54. Walks and paces constantly									
55. Very suspicious/paranoid									
56. Has delusional ideas									
57. Has hallucinations									
58. Sexually inappropriate									

OTHER

59.									
60.									
61.									
62.									
63.									

Using the Personal/Social Support Resources

Family members often become isolated in caregiving; however, this is not inevitable. Contact with the outside world can be maintained. As stress and pressures of caregiving build, it is difficult to think of who can help. Thus it is a good idea to identify persons to call on for assistance before you become overwhelmed by too many demands and have no time to think.

First, it is helpful to evaluate the supports within the family and neighborhood. As independent people, many caregivers like to think they can always take care of themselves, but constant caregiving can change things. They may need much more support and help; That is when caregivers can turn to family, friends, neighbors, church members, or professionals for help.

We have found in our work that it is often difficult initially for caregivers to complete this form. Too often, only one person is the support for all areas covered by the questions. It is important for others to be considered as backup resources and for the caregiver to begin to rely on at least one or two people to cover some of the areas. Family support groups can be important resources.

Some of the questions point to a need for a more immediate source of security. For example, when the caregiver is frightened, he or she needs to talk to someone quickly. If the behavior of the relative is threatening, the caregiver may want to call the doctor or mental health professional. If the caregiver suspects a burglar is in the house, he or she must call the police.

Different resources may be more appropriate for different questions. Caregivers are encouraged to use this form to examine closely their total support network. A confidant is a valuable resource, but other personal resources may need to be developed.

PERSONAL/SOCIAL SUPPORT RESOURCES

NAME: _____ DATE: _____

Using your own situation, check the most appropriate Personal/Social Supports to the right of each question. Try to check at least 3.

	Yourself	Spouse	Children	Other Family	Friends	Neighbors	Church	Pastor/Priest	Doctor	Other Professional	Support Group	Agency Staff	Other
1. Who can you count on for transportation?													
2. Who can you count on for financial help/decisions?													
3. Who helps most with household chores?													
4. Who can you count on to get to appointments?													
5. Who do you enjoy doing things with during the week?													
6. Who can you count on in time of crisis?													
7. Who can you count on when you're physically sick?													
8. Who can you count on to console you when you're very upset?													
9. Who would you seek out when you're frightened?													
10. Who would you talk to when you're lonely?													
11. When you need to talk, who can you count on to listen?													
12. With whom can you really be yourself?													
13. Who do you trust completely?													
14. Who do you feel really appreciates you as a person?													
15. With whom do you have the most frequent contact?													
16. Whose advice are you most likely to accept?													
17. Who supports your independence the most?													

Using your own situation, check the most appropriate Personal/Social Supports to the right of each question. Try to check at least 3.

	Yourself	Spouse	Children	Other Family	Friends	Neighbors	Church	Pastor/Priest	Doctor	Other Professional	Support Group	Agency Staff	Other
18. Who seems to understand you best?													
19. Who helps you to be honest with yourself?													
20. Who helps you keep a positive outlook?													
21. Who do you enjoy being with the most?													
22. Who best understands your current situation?													
23. Who helps you work out your problems most?													
24. Who could temporarily take your place in caregiving?													
25. Who do you trust regarding legal matters?													
26. Who can you talk to about family problems?													

In-Home Care List

This form may be used by family members to determine how much assistance their relatives actually need to perform activities of daily living. Realistic expectations can develop, and this information can be communicated to other persons who help with caregiving. Alzheimer's patients should be encouraged to do what they can for themselves; family members must avoid doing things for them unnecessarily.

Some persons with Alzheimer's disease still live alone. In these cases, the "In-Home Care List" will help family members to determine how much assistance the person needs.

Nursing homes can use this form to get a better idea of how much assistance the resident will require in daily living activities, socialization, and leisure/recreational activities. This scale is a planning, communication, and monitoring tool. Other professionals may use it to help families secure appropriate community resources.

For each behavior check the category that best describes how it occurs. For example, for the behavior to occur appropriately or as one desires, verbal assistance, physical assistance, or complete supervision may be necessary. On the other hand there may be no need for assistance of any kind for the behavior to occur as desired on a regular basis. In some cases the behavior may not be carried out as desired or appropriately even with complete supervision. In that case one should check that the behavior does not occur appropriately. Put NA for "not applicable" when that behavior does not apply.

Definitions

Without assistance: The behavior occurs appropriately with no assistance or corrective devices (e.g., glasses, hearing aid, walker, etc.).

With verbal assistance: The behavior occurs appropriately or as desired with *only* verbal cues, reminders, instructions, directions, and so forth.

With physical assistance: Verbal assistance is not enough; physical assistance is required for the behavior to occur appropriately; the caregiver physically assists or does for the person; glasses and other adaptive devices represent physical assistance.

With total supervision: The behavior occurs only if totally supervised. Both verbal and physical assistance may be necessary as part of the supervision.

Behavior does not occur appropriately: The behavior does not occur as desired even with assistance and supervision.

IN-HOME CARE LIST

NAME: _____   DATE: _____

	Behavior Occurs Appropriately:			Behavior Does Not Occur Appropriately
	Without Assistance	W/Verbal Assistance	W/Physical Assistance	W/Total Supervision	

I. Activities of Daily Living

Basic

A. Dresses self
B. Bathes regularly
C. Eats regular meals
D. Takes prescribed medication
E. Takes over-the-counter medications
F. Uses bathroom as necessary
G. Grooms self regularly
H. Wears clean clothing

Advanced

A. Prepares meals
B. Does food shopping
C. Pays bills
D. Uses telephone
E. Uses stove safely
F. Follows medical advice
G. Handles money
H. Washes clothes
I. Keeps house clean

J. Follows daily routines
K. Wears suitable clothing for weather
L. Seeks help when needed
M. Drives car
N. Has regular contact with doctor

II. Socialization

A. Leaves house for social activities
B. Good interaction with friends, neighbors
C. Good interaction with spouse
D. Good interaction with other family
E. Expresses self
F. Understands what others say
G. Recognizes familiar people
H. Generally gets along with people

III. Leisure Activities

A. Follows specific instructions
B. Walks in yard
C. Walks in neighborhood
D. Reads newspaper
E. Watches TV
F. Plays games
G. Looks at magazines
H. Enjoys gardening
I. Listens to music
J. Enjoys arts and crafts
K. Does exercise

OTHER:

Care Management Stress

This form can be useful for the family caregiver and professionals involved with the caregiver and the Alzheimer's patient. It is another approach to problem solving and making changes in the caregiver situation. Some changes must occur as a result of psychological adjustment, but family support and outside resources can help. For example, when it is hard to accept the diagnosis of Alzheimer's, the caregiver needs time to adjust and plenty of information in order to understand what lies ahead for both patient and caregiver. For a caregiver who experiences frequent financial problems, family meetings to discuss possibilities and an investigation of community resources may prove helpful.

When a caregiver often feels isolated and abandoned, other people showing their care and concern can help. Other statements reflect the caregiver's response to frequent stress. Another cluster of statements may suggest depression or other adjustment problems that may require professional treatment. For example, being overly upset or fatigued, sleeping poorly, or feeling nervous, all suggest the need for more support, counseling, and perhaps treatment for the caregiver.

Family problems or feelings of estrangement may be evident if statements concerning family are rated frequently. These kinds of problems may require counseling or other approaches to bring the family back together or to develop ways to accept dissenting family views.

This stress scale can assist caregivers in assessing how they are coping over the duration of the caregiving experience.

CARE MANAGEMENT STRESS

CAREGIVER: _____ DATE: _____ AGE: _____

CLIENT: _____ AGE: _____ DURATION OF CAREGIVING: _____

Please check a response for each.

	NEVER	RARELY	SOMETIMES	FREQUENTLY	NEARLY ALWAYS
1. I'm uncomfortable leaving my relative alone.					
2. Worries bother me a lot.					
3. I get tired and worn out doing everything.					
4. Family fail to understand what I'm experiencing.					
5. Everyone fails to appreciate what is happening.					
6. Family members could help a lot more.					
7. I'd like to see friends more.					
8. My relative's behavior frightens me.					
9. It's hard now to accept this diagnosis.					
10. It's hard for my family to accept this diagnosis.					
11. I'm feeling more tense and nervous.					
12. I have a lot of financial concerns.					
13. My relative asks too much of me.					
14. I feel abandoned by doctors/professionals.					
15. I feel my health is suffering because of this.					
16. Decisions are hard for me to make.					
17. I feel I need more rest and sleep.					
18. Family members think I should do more.					
19. I feel I need more privacy.					
20. I'm unable to get out to do what I need to.					
21. I'm embarrassed by my relative's behavior.					
22. I get easily upset with my relative.					
23. I feel I need more help.					
24. I feel I'm getting isolated.					
25. I'm afraid of what the future will be.					

Staff Stress Measure

This form is designed for use in nursing homes and day programs that care for Alzheimer's patients. For persons in supervisory and staff development positions, it can be useful in developing training programs and in working individually with employees. Direct care staff have the most contact with the Alzheimer's patient; therefore, they need a better understanding of the illness, how to deal with the behavior, and how to cope with this behavior emotionally. They need skills and sensitivity.

These staff in an open and supportive learning environment can be open and honest about their frustration and fears. They can also be receptive to suggestions when they begin to understand that the behavior of brain-impaired individuals can be more predictable and manageable.

STAFF STRESS MEASURE
DEMENTIA CARE

All statements below reflect feelings and beliefs that apply to work with residents who have Alzheimer's disease or a similar degenerative dementia. For each statement check how often you are affected in such a way.

	Rarely	Sometimes	Frequently	Nearly Always
1. Their forgetfulness really gets on my nerves.				
2. I believe these residents should do more for themselves.				
3. I'm afraid these residents will get violent and hurt someone.				
4. I get tired of repeating things to them so much.				
5. Their families just don't appreciate what we do for these people.				
6. Their babbling and rambling speech gets on my nerves.				
7. It's very hard for me to communicate with these people.				
8. I get mad when they deny problems and blame others for things.				
9. I really get tired working with these residents.				
10. It's hard to accept what is happening to these residents.				
11. I get frustrated and angry working with these people.				
12. I think more medication would make it easier to help them.				
13. I have trouble talking to their families.				
14. I take my work with them home with me.				
15. I feel these residents should appreciate our help more.				
16. It worries me these people will wander off.				
17. I feel it takes too long to do things for them.				
18. It bothers me how helpless these residents become.				
19. I believe we should have more training to work with them.				
20. It's difficult to explain their behavior to other residents or families.				

SERVICE/RESOURCE WORKSHEET
Example

Name of agency: *Home Health Care*

Type of service/resource needed: *Supervision of Alzheimer's patient in the home and assistance with basic personal care (bathing)*

What the service/resource will accomplish: *give caregiver time to get away, and do necessary errands, visit, shop*

Agency/individual providing service—contact person: *Home Health Care: Jodie Smith*

Eligibility requirements (income, age, geographic): *none for this type of service*

Fees/cost of service: *$5.00 an hour for 10 hours*

Projected cost of service over time: *about $200.00 a month times 12 months*

Sliding scale for fee structure: *none—different hourly rates for total monthly hours*

Insurance coverage—how much, how long: *none, unless nursing care needed*

In-home and/or office services: *All services provided in the home*

Benefit of service to family: *gives caregiver a break, time to do other things*

Other services provided by this agency: *Agency also has medical equipment, nursing services, occupational, physical, and speech therapists*

Providers recommended by professionals and/or friends: *This agency and Home Help Health Care (which is $8.00 an hour regardless)*

APPENDIX B

SELF-HELP GROUPS AND ORGANIZATIONS THAT CAN HELP

U.S. Department of Health and Human Services
Alzheimer's Disease Education and Referral Center, P.O. Box 8250, Silver Spring, MD 20907-8250, 800-438-4380

Alzheimer's Association

A network of self-support groups exists through the Alzheimer's Association. Groups that have just become affiliated may not be listed here. There are also local support groups in some areas that are not affiliated with the Alzheimer's Association. These groups may be helpful to the caregiver. To find out about a support group in your area, contact the Area Agency on Aging or the Information and Referral Program. The Alzheimer's Association will have information about affiliated groups, and information about the disease and caregiving.

National Office—Alzheimer's Association, 919 N. Michigan Ave., Suite 1000, Chicago, IL 60611-1676, 312-335-8700

The Alzheimer's Association has an Information and Referral Service Line. Through it you can locate the support group nearest you. Call: 800-272-3900.

American Health Assistance Foundation

The American Health Assistance Foundation (AHAF) is devoted to funding scientific research on Alzheimer's disease as well as other age-related and degenerative diseases. AHAF's Alzheimer's Family Relief Program provides direct emergency financial assistance to Alzheimer's disease victims and caregivers when no other means are available. The Foundation also offers free educational materials on Alzheimer's disease upon request.

The American Health Assistance Foundation, 15825 Shady Grove Road, Suite 140, Rockville, MD 20850, 301-948-3244 or 800-437-2423.

Area Agencies on Aging

Area Agencies on Aging carry out implementations of programs for older persons that are indicated by the Older American's Act. The Administration on Aging has this responsibility at the federal level. Area Agencies on Aging are a local extension of the federal agency. Usually there is a state Department on Aging that governs Area Agencies on Aging for each state. The reader may call the State Department to determine what Area Agency on Aging covers his particular location. State Departments or Area Agencies on Aging can also provide information concerning Nursing Home Ombudsman Programs.

Administration on Aging
330 Independence Avenue
Washington, DC 20201
General Information: 202-472-7257

Alabama

Commission on Aging, 136 Catoma St., 2nd Floor, Montgomery, AL 36130; 205-242-5743

Alaska

Older Alaskans Commission, Department of Administration, Pouch C-MS-0209, Juneau, AK 99811; 907-465-3250

Arizona

Office on Aging and Adult Administration, Department of Economic Security, 1400 West Washington Street, Phoenix, AZ 85007; 602-255-3596

Arkansas

Division of Aging and Adult Services, Arkansas Department of Human Services, P.O. Box 1417, Slot 1412, 7th and Main Sts., Little Rock, AR 72201; 501-682-2441

California

Department of Aging, 1600 K Street, Sacramento, CA 95814; 96-322-5290

Colorado

Aging and Adult Services Division, Department of Social Services, 1575 Sherman St., 10th Floor, Denver, CO 80203-1714; 303-866-3851

Connecticut

Department on Aging, 175 Main Street, Hartford, CT 06106; 203-566-3238

Delaware

Department of Health and Social Services, Division of Aging, 1901 North Dupont Highway, New Castle, DE 19720; 302-421-6791

District of Columbia

Office of Aging, 1424 K Street, N.W., Washington, DC 20005; 202-724-5626

Florida

Program Office of Aging and Adult Services, Department of Health and Rehabilitative Services, 1317 Winewood Boulevard, Tallahassee, FL 32301; 904-488-8922

Georgia

Office of Aging, 878 Peachtree Street, N.E., Room 632, Atlanta, GA 30309; 404-894-5333

Hawaii

Executive Office on Aging, Office of the Governor, State of Hawaii, Room 241, 335 Merchant Street, Honolulu, HI 96813; 808-548-2593

Idaho

Idaho Office on Aging, Statehouse Room 114, Boise, ID 83720; 208-334-3833

Illinois

Illinois Department on Aging, 421 East Capitol Avenue, Springfield, IL 62701; 217-785-2870

Indiana

Division of Aging Services, Department of Human Services, 251 North Illinois Street, P.O. Box 7083, Indianapolis, IN 46207-8083; 317-232-7020

Iowa

Department of Elder Affairs, Suite 236, Jewett Building, 914 Grand Avenue, Des Moines, IA 50319; 515-281-5187

Kansas

Kansas Department of Aging, Docking State Office Building, 122-S, 915 S.W. Harrison, Topeka, KS 66612-1500; 913-296-4986

Kentucky

Kentucky Division of Aging Services, Cabinet for Human Resources, CHR Building-6th West, 275 East Main Street, Frankfort, KY 40621; 502-564-6930

Louisiana

Louisiana Office of Elderly Affairs, 4550 North Blvd. P.O. Box 80374, Baton Rouge, LA 70806; 504-925-1700

Maine

Bureau of Elder and Adult Services, Department of Human Services, State House Station 11, Augusta, ME 04333; 207-289-2561

Maryland

Maryland Office on Aging, State Office Building, 301 West Preston Street, Room 1004, Baltimore, MD 21201; 301-225-1100

Massachusetts

Executive Office of Elder Affairs, 38 Chauncey Street, Boston, MA 02111; 617-727-7750

Michigan

Michigan Office of Services to the Aging, 300 East Michigan, P.O. Box 30026, Lansing, MI 48909; 517-373-8230

Minnesota

Minnesota Board on Aging, Human Services Building, 4th Floor, 444 Lafayette Rd., St. Paul, MN 55155-3843; 612-296-2770

Mississippi

Mississippi Council on Aging, Division of Aging and Adult Services, 421 W. Pascagoula St., Jackson, MS 39203; 601-949-2070

Missouri

Division on Aging, Department of Social Services, P.O. Box 1337, 2701 West Main Street, Jefferson City, MO 65102; 314-751-3082

Montana

Governor's Office on Aging, State Capitol Building, Capitol Station, Helena, MT 59620; 406-444-3111

Nebraska

Nebraska Department on Aging, P.O. Box 95044, 301 Centennial Mall South, Lincoln, NE 68509; 402-471-2306

Nevada

Division of Aging Services, Department of Human Resources, 340 N. 11th St., Las Vegas, NV 89101; 702-486-3545

New Hampshire

Division of Elderly and Adult Services, 6 Hazen Dr., Concord, NH 03301-6501; 603-271-4680

New Jersey

Division on Aging, Department of Community Affairs, CN807, S. Broad and Front Sts., West State Street, Trenton, NJ 00625-0807; 609-292-4833

New Mexico

New Mexico State Agency on Aging, La Villa Rivera Building, 4th Floor, 224 East Palace Avenue, Santa Fe, NM 87501; 505-827-7640

New York

Office for the Aging, New York State Plaza, Agency Building 2, Albany, NY 12223; 518-474-4425

North Carolina

Division on Aging, 693 Palmer Dr., Raleigh, NC 27603; 919-733-3983

North Dakota

Aging Services, Department of Human Services, State Capital Building, Bismark, MD 58505; 701-224-2577

Ohio

Ohio Department on Aging, Ninth Floor, 50 West Broad Street, Columbus, OH 43266-0501; 614-466-5500

Oklahoma

Aging Services Division, Department of Human Services, P.O. Box 25352, Oklahoma City, OK 73125; 405-521-2281

Oregon

Senior Services Division, Human Resources Department, 313 Public Services Building, Salem, OR 97310; 503-378-4728

Pennsylvania

Pennsylvania Department of Aging, 231 State Street, Harrisburg, PA 17101-1195; 717-783-1550

Rhode Island

Department of Elderly Affairs, 160 Pine St., Providence, RI 02903-3708; 401-277-2858

South Carolina

South Carolina Commission of Aging, 400 Arbor Lake Dr., Suite B-500, Columbia, SC 29223; 803-735-0210

South Dakota

Office of Adult Services and Aging, Richard F. Kneip Building, 700 North Illinois Street, Pierre, SD 57501; 605-773-3656

Tennessee

Tennessee Commission on Aging, Suite 201, 706 Church Street, Nashville, TN 37219-5573; 615-741-2056

Texas

Texas Department of Aging, P.O. Box 12786, Capital Station, 1949 IH 35 South, Austin, TX 78741-3702; 512-444-2727

Utah

Division of Aging and Adult Services, Department of Social Services, 120 North-200 West, Box 45500, Salt Lake City, UT 84145-0500; 801-533-3910

Vermont

Department of Rehabilitation and Aging, 103 South Main Street, Waterbury, VT 05676; 802-241-2400

Virginia

Virginia Department on Aging, 700 Centre, 10th Floor, 700 E. Franklin St., Richmond, VA 23219-2327; 804-225-2271

Washington

Aging and Adult Services Administration, Department of Social and Health Services, OB-44B, Olympia, WA 98504; 206-586-3768

West Virginia

Commission on Aging, Holly Grove-State Capitol, Charleston, WV 25305; 304-348-3317

Wisconsin

Bureau of Aging, Division of Community Services, 217 S. Hamilton St., Suite 300, Madison, WI 53707; 608-266-2536

Wyoming

Commission on Aging, Room 139, Hathaway Building, Cheyenne, WY 82002-0710; 307-777-7986

BIBLIOGRAPHY

Agbayewa, O.M. "Earlier Psychiatric Morbidity in Patients with Alzheimer's Disease." *JAGS, 34* (1986):561–564.

Aisen, P., and Davis, K. "Inflammatory Mechanisms in Alzheimer's Disease: Implications for Therapy." *American Journal of Psychiatry, 151* (1994):1105–1113.1.

Beaumont, J.G. *Introduction to Neuropsychology.* New York: The Gullford Press, 1983.

Blazer, D. "Evaluating the Family of the Elderly Patient." *A Family Approach to Health Care of the Elderly,* edited by Blazer, D., and Siegler, I., 13–32. Menlo Park, CA: Addison–Wesley, 1984.

Bloom, T.E. et al. *Brain, Mind, and Behavior.* New York: W.H. Freeman and Company, 1985.

Bondareff, W. "Age and Alzheimer's Disease." *The Lancet* (June 25, 1983):1447.

Bondareff, W. "Biomedical Perspective of Alzheimer's Disease and Dementia in the Elderly." In *The Dementias: Policy and Management,* edited by Gilhooly M.L.M. et al., 13–37. New Jersey: Prentice-Hall, 1986.

Breitner, J. "Inflammatory Processes and Anti-inflammatory Drugs in Alzheimer's Disease: A Current Appraisal." *Neurobiology of Aging, 17* (1996):789–794.

Breitner, J., and Gau, B. "Inverse Association of Anti-Inflammatory Treatments and Alzheimer's Disease: Initial Results of a Co-Twin Study." *Neurology, 44* (1994):227:232.

Brun, A. "An Overview of Light and Electron Microscopic Changes." In *Alzheimer's Disease: The Standard Reference,* edited by Reisberg, B., 37–48. New York: The Free Press, 1983.

Bruno, G. et al. "Muscarinic Agonist Therapy of Alzheimer's Disease." *Arch. Neurol., 43* (1986):459–661.

Carlsson, A. "Changes in Neurotransmitter Systems in the Aging Brain and in Alzheimer's Disease." In *Alzheimer's Disease: The Standard Reference,* edited by Reisberg, B., 100–106. New York: The Free Press, 1983.

Cohen, D., and Eisdorfer, C. *The Loss of Self: A Family Resource for the Care of Alzheimer's Disease and Related Disorders.* New York: W.W. Norton and Company, 1986.

Cohen, S., and Whiteford, W. *Caregiving with Grace.* (Video Production) Baltimore Life Care, Inc. 1987.

Conley, Charles, M.D. Personal communication with author, July, 1987.

Cooper, S.J. "Drug Treatments, Neurochemical Change and Human Memory Impairment." In *Clinical Management of Memory Problems,* edited by Wilson, Barbara, and Moffat, Nick, 132–147. London: Aspen Publication, 1984,

Corder, E. et al. "Gene Dose of Apolipoprotein E Type 4 Allele and the Risk of Alzheimer's Disease in Late-Onset Families." *Science, 261* (1993):921–923.

Coyle, J.T. et al. "Alzheimer's Disease: A Disorder of Cortical Cholinergic Innerva-
tion." *Science, 219* (1983): 1184–1189.

Cummings, J.L., and Benson, D.F. *Dementia: A Clinical Approach.* Boston: Butter-
worths, 1983, 35–167.

Cummings, J.L., and Benson, D.F. "Subcortical Dementia." *Arch. Neurol., 41*
(1984):874–879.

Davies, P., and Wolozin, B.L. "Recent Advances in the Neurochemistry of
Alzheimer's Disease." *J. Clin. Psychiatry, 48* (1987):23–30.

Davies, K.L. et al. "Cholinergic Treatment in Alzheimer's Disease: Implications for
Future Research." In *Alzheimer's Disease: A Report of Progress in Research*
(Aging, Vol. 19), edited by Corkin, S. et al., 483–494. New York: Raven Press,
1982.

DeKosky, S. "Advances in the Biology of Alzheimer's Disease." In *The Dementias:*
Diagnosis, Management and Research, edited by Weiner, M. 313–330. Washington, D.C.: American Psychiatric Press, 1996.

Diagnostic and Statistical Manual of Mental Disorders, 4th Edition. 1994. Washington, D.C.: American Psychiatric Association.

Diagnostic and Statistical Manual of Mental Disorders, 3rd Edition. 1980. Washington, D.C.: American Psychiatric Association.

Dysken, M.W. "A Review of Recent Clinical Trials in the Treatment of Alzheimer's
Dementia." *Psychiatric Annals, 17* (1987):178–191.

Editorial. "Cholinergic Treatment in Alzheimer's Disease: Encouraging Results." *The*
Lancet (Jan. 17, 1987):139–141.

Edye, D., and Rich, J. *Psychological Distress in Aging: A Family Management*
Model. Rockville, Maryland: Aspen Publication, 1983.

Etienne, P. "Treatment of Alzheimer's Disease with Lecithin." In *Alzheimer's Disease: The Standard Reference,* edited by Reisberg, B., 353–354. New York: The
Free Press, 1983.

Ferris, S.H. "Neuropeptides in the Treatment of Alzheimer's Disease." In *Alzheimer's*
Disease: The Standard Reference, edited by Reisberg, B., 369–373. New York:
The Free Press, 1983.

Fine, A. "Transplantation in the Central Nervous System." *Scien. Amer., 255*
(1986):52–59.

Fovall, P., Dysken, M.W., and Davis, J.M. "Treatment of Alzheimer's Disease with
Choline Salts." In *Alzheimer's Disease: The Standard Reference,* edited by Reisberg, B., 346–353. New York: The Free Press, 1983.

Gage, F.H. et al. "Intrahippocampal Septal Grafts Ameliorate Learning Impairments
in Aged Rats." *Science,* (1984):533–536.

Gallagher, D., Rose, J., Rivera, P., Lovett, S., and Thompson, L. "Prevalence of Depression in Family Caregivers." *Gerontologist, 29* (1989):449–456.

Gash, D.M. et al. "Neuronal Transplantation: A Review of Recent Developments
and Potential Applications to the Aged Brain." *Neurobiology of Aging,*
6 (1985):131–150.

Goldsmith, M.F. "Attempts to Vanquish Alzheimer's Disease Intensify, Take New
Paths." *JAMA, 251* (1984):1805–1807, 1811–1812.

Gottfries, C.G. "Neurotransmitters in the brains of patients with dementia disorders."
DMB, Gerontology, 1 (1985):44–47.

Gwyther, L. "Clinician and Family: A Partnership for Support." In *Dementia Care:*
Patient, Family, and Community, edited by Mace, N., 193–230. Baltimore: Johns
Hopkins University Press, 1990.

Gwyther, L. "Letting Go: Separation—Individuation in a Wife of an Alzheimer's
Patient." *Gerontologist, 30* (1990):698–702.

Henderson, V. et al. "Estrogen Replacement Therapy in Older Women." *Achives of Neurology, 51* (1994):896–900.

Henig, R. *The Myth of Senility: Misconceptions about the Brain and Aging.* Doubleday: Anchor Press, 1981.

Henry, J.P. "Relation of Psychosocial Factors to the Senile Dementias." In *The Dementias: Policy and Management,* edited by Gilhooly, M.L. et al., 38–65. New Jersey: Prentice-Hall, 1986.

Heston, L.L. *Alzheimer's Disease and Related Disorders Association Newsletter, 5* (Summer 1985).

Heston, L.L., and White, J. *Dementia: A Practical Guide to Alzheimer's Disease and Related Disorders.* New York: W.H. Freeman and Co., 1983.

Hill, P.H., and Henderson, V. "Estrogen Deficiency and Risk of Alzheimer's Disease in Women." *American Journal of Epidemiology, 140* (1994):256–261.

Hyman, B.T. et al. "Alzheimer's Disease: Cell-specific Pathology Isolates the Hippocampal Formation." *Science, 225* (1984):1168–1170.

Jenike, M.A. et al. "Combination Therapy with Lecithin and Ergoloid Mesylates for Alzheimer's Disease." *J. Am. Psychiatry, 47* (1986):249–251.

Katzman, R. "Alzheimer's Disease." *N. Engl. J. Med., 314* (1986):964–973.

Katzman, R. "Current Research on Alzheimer's Disease in a Historical Perspective." In *Alzheimer's Disease: Cause(s), Diagnosis, Treatment and Care,* edited by Khachaturian, Z., and Radebaugh, T., 15–29. New York: CRC Press, 1996.

Katzman, R. "The Prevalence and Malignancy of Alzheimer's Disease; A Major Killer." *Archives of Neurology, 33* (1976):217.

Kaye, W.H. et al. "Cognitive Effects of Cholinergic and Vasopressin-like Agents in Patients with Primary Degenerative Dementia." In *Alzheimer's Disease: A Report of Progress in Research (Aging,* Vol. 19), edited by Corkin, S. et al., 433–422. New York: Raven Press, 1982.

Kaye, W.H., Sitaram, N. et al. "Modest Facilitation of Memory in Dementia with Combined Lecithin and Anticholinesterase Treatment." *Biol. Psychiatry, 17* (1982):275–280.

Kemper, T. "Neuroanatomical and Neuropathological Changes in Normal Aging and in Dementia."In *Clinical Neurology of Aging,* edited by Albert, M. New York: Oxford University Press, 1984.

Kolb, B., and Whishaw, I. *Fundamentals of Human Neuropsychology.* San Francisco: W.H. Freeman and Co., 1980.

Kübler-Ross, E. *On Death and Dying.* New York: Macmillan, 1969, 38–137.

Lawton, M.P. "Environmental Approaches to Research and Treatment of Alzheimer's Disease." In *Alzheimer's Disease Treatment and Family Stress: Directions for Research.* 340–362. U.S. Department of Health and Human Services. DHHS Publication No. (ADM) 89–1569, 1989.

Lewin, L., and Lundervold, D. "Behavioral Analysis of Separation—Individuation Conflict in the Spouse of an Alzeimer's Disease Patient." *Gerontologist, 30* (1990):703–705.

Lichtenberg, P., and Barth, J. "The Dynamic Process of Caregiving in Elderly Spouses: A Look at Longitudinal Case Reports." *Clinical Gerontologist, 9* (1989):31–44.

McDuff, T., and Sumi, S.M. "Subcortical Degeneration in Alzheimer's Disease." *Neuro., 35* (1985):123–126.

McGreer, P., and McGreer, E. "Neuroimmune Mechanisms in the Pathogenesis of Alzheimer's Disease." In *Alzheimer's Disease: Cause(s), Diagnosis, Treatment and Care,* edited by Khachaturian, Z., and Radebaugh, T., 217–225. New York: CRC Press, 1996.

Mace, N. "The Management of Problem Behaviors." In *Dementia Care: Patient, Family, and Community,* edited by Mace, N., 74–112. Baltimore: Johns Hopkins University Press, 1990.

Mace, N., and Rabins, P. *The 36-Hour Day.* Rev. Ed. Baltimore: Johns Hopkins University Press, 1991.

Madrazo, I. et al. "Open Microsurgical Autograft of Adrenal Medulla to the Right Caudate Nucleus in Two Patients with Intractable Parkinson's Disease." *N. Engl. J. Med., 316* (1987):831–834.

Markesbery, W. "Trace Elements in Alzheimer's Disease." In *Alzheimer's Disease: Cause(s), Diagnosis, Treatment and Care,* edited by Khachaturian, Z., and Radebaugh, T., 233–236. New York: CRC Press, 1996.

Mayeux, R. et al. "Heterogeneity in Dementia of the Alzheimer-type: Evidence of Subgroups." *Neuro., 35* (1985):453–461.

Mayeux, R. "Putative Risk Factors for Alzheimer's Disease." In *Alzheimer's Disease: Cause(s), Diagnosis, Treatment and Care,* edited by Khachaturian, Z., and Radebaugh, T., 39–49. New York: CRC Press, 1996.

Merz, B. "Adrenal-to-Brain Transplants Improve the Prognosis for Parkinson's Disease." *JAMA, 257* (1987):2691–2692.

Miller, J. "Family Support of the Elderly." *Aging and Health Promotion,* Collected works by Wells, T., Rockville, MD: Aspen Publication, 1982.

Mohs, R.C., and Davis, B.M. et al. "Clinical Studies of the Cholinergic Deficit in Alzheimer's Disease." *JAGS, 33* (1985):749–757.

Moore, R.Y. "Parkinson's Disease—A New Therapy?" *N. Engl. J. Med., 316* (1987):872–873.

Nee, L.E. et al. "A Family with Histologically Confirmed Alzheimer's Disease." *Arch. Neurol., 40* (1983):203–208.

Oliver, R., and Bock, F. "Alleviating the Distress of Caregivers of Alzheimer's Disease Patients: A Rational-Emotive Therapy Model." *Clinical Gerontology, 3* (1985):4.

Pearlin, L. et al. "Caregiving and the Stress Process: An Overview of Concepts and Their Measures." *Gerontologist, 30* (1990):583–594.

Pericak-Vance et al. "Linkage Studies in Familial Alzheimer's Disease: Evidence for Chromosome 19 Linkage." *American Journal of Human Genetics, 48* (1991):1034–1050.

Perry, E.K., and Perry, R.H. "A Review of Neuropathological and Neurochemical Correlates of Alzheimer's Disease." *DMB, Gerontology, 1* (1985):27–34.

Peskind, E. "Neurobiology of Alzheimer's Disease." *Journal of Clinical Psychiatry, 57* (Supplement) (1996):5–8.

Peters, B.H., and Levin, H.S. "Chronic Oral Physostigmine and Lecithin Administration in Memory Disorders of Aging." In *Alzheimer's Disease: A Report of Progress in Research (Aging,* Vol. 19), edited by Corkin, S. et al., 421–426. New York: Ravin Press, 1982.

Pollen, D. *Hannah's Heirs: The Quest for the Genetic Origins of Alzheimer's Disease.* New York: Oxford University Press, 1996.

Powell, L., and Courtice, K. *Alzheimer's Disease: A Guide for Families.* Reading, Massachusetts: Addison-Wesley Publishing Co., 1983.

Prien, R.F. "Psychostimulants in the Treatment of Senile Dementia." In *Alzheimer's Disease: The Standard Reference,* edited by Reisberg, B., 381–386. New York: The Free Press, 1983.

Pruchno, R., and Resch, N. "Husbands and Wives as Caregivers: Antecedents of Depression and Burden." *Gerontologist, 29* (1989):159–165.

Prusiner, S.B. "Some Speculations about Prions, Amyloid, and Alzheimer's Disease." *N. Engl. J. Med., 310* (1984):661–663.

Rando, Therese. *Grief, Dying, and Death: Clinical Interventions for Caregivers.* Champaign, IL: Research Press, 1984.

Reisberg, B. *A Guide to Alzheimer's Disease: For Families, Spouses and Friends.* New York: The Free Press, 1981.

Reisberg, B. (ed.) Alzheimer's Disease: The Standard Reference. New York: The Free Press, 1983.

Reisberg, B. et al. "Signs, Symptoms and Course of Age-associated Cognitive Decline." In *Alzheimer's Disease: A Report of Progress in Research (Aging,* Vol. 19), edited by Corkin, S. et al., 177–182. New York: Raven Press, 1982.

Reisberg, B. et al. "Effects of Naloxone in Senile Dementia." *N. Engl. J. Med., 308* (1983):721–722.

Restak, Richard M. *The Brain.* New York: Bantam Books; 1984, 10–14, 338–342.

Rogers, J. et al. "Immune-Related Mechanisms of Alzheimer's Disease Pathogenesis." In *Alzheimer's Disease: New Treatment Strategies,* edited by Khachaturian, Z., and Blass, J., 147–163. New York: Marcel Dekker, 1992.

Rose, J., and DelMaestro, S. "Separation—Individuation Conflict as a Model for Understanding Distressed Caregivers: Psychodynamic and Cognitive Case Studies." *Gerontologist, 30* (1990):693–697.

Rosenberg, G.S. et al. "Pharmacologic Treatment of Alzheimer's Disease: An Overview." In *Alzheimer's Disease: The Standard Reference,* edited by Reisberg, B., 329–339. New York: The Free Press, 1983.

Roses, A. "The Metabolism of Apolipoprotein E and the Alzheimer's Diseases." In *Alzheimer's Disease: Cause(s), Diagnosis, Treatment and Care,* edited by Khachaturian, Z., and Radebaugh, T., 207–216. New York: CRC Press, 1996.

Roses, A. et al. "Clinical Application of Apolipoprotein E Genotyping to Alzheimer's Disease." *The Lancet, 343* (1994):1564–1565.

Sano, M. et al. "A Controlled Trial of Selegiline, Alpha-Tocopherol, or Both as Treatment for Alzheimer's Disease." *New England Journal of Medicine, 336* (1997):1216–1222.

Schmeck, Harold. "Blood Abnormality May Predict Alzheimer's." *The New York Times* (October 29, 1987).

Schneck, M.K. "Nootropics." In *Alzheimer's Disease: The Standard Reference,* edited by Reisberg, B., 362–268. New York: The Free Press, 1983.

Selkoe, D.J. et al. "Conservation of Brain Amyloid Proteins in Aged Mammals and Humans with Alzheimer's Disease." *Science, 235* (1987):873–877.

Shihabuddin, L., and Davis, K. "Treatment of Alzheimer's Disease." In *Alzheimer's Disease: Cause(s), Diagnosis, Treatment and Care,* edited by Khachaturian, Z., and Radebaugh, T., 257–274. New York: CRC Press, 1996.

Shomaker, D. "Problematic Behavior and the Alzheimer's Patient: Retrospection as a Method of Understanding and Counseling." *Gerontologist, 27* (1987):370–375.

Shore, P., and Wyatt, R.J. "Aluminum and Alzheimer's Disease." *J. Nervous Ment. Disease, 171* (1983):353–558.

Siegler, I., and Hyer, L. "Common Crises in the Family Life of Older Persons." *A Family Approach to Health Care of the Elderly,* Edited by Blazer, D. and Siegler, I., 33–50. Menlo Park, CA: Addison-Wesley, 1984.

Simpkins, J. et al. "The Potential Role for Estrogen Replacement Therapy in Treatment of the Cognitive Decline and Neurogeneration Associated with Alzheimer's Disease." *Neurobiology of Aging, 15* (Supple 2) (1994):S195–S197.

Sitaram, N. et al. "Combination Treatment of Alzheimer's Dementia." In *Alzheimer's Disease: The Standard Reference,* edited by Reisberg, B., 355–361. New York: The Free Press, 1983.

Stearn, R., and Davis, K. "Research in Treating Cognitive Impairment in Alzheimer's

Disease." In *The Dementias: Diagnosis, Management, and Research* (2nd Edition), edited by Weiner, M., 331–353. Washington, D.C.: American Psychiatric Press, 1996.

Stephenson, J. "Researchers Find Evidence of a New Gene for Late-Onset Alzheimer's Disease." *JAMA, 277* (1997):775.

Stewart, W. "Risk of Alzheimer's Disease and Duration of NSAID Use." *Neurology, 48* (1997): 626–632.

Tagliavini, F., and Pilleri, G. "Neuronal Counts in Basal Nucleus of Meynert in Alzheimer's Disease." *The Lancet* (Feb. 26, 1983):469–470.

Tamminga, N.L. et al. "Alzheimer's Disease: Low Cerebral Somatostatin Levels Correlate with Impaired Cognitive Function and Cortical Metabolism." *Neurology, 37* (1987):161–165.

Tang, M-X. et al. "Effect of Estrogen During Menopause on Risk and Age at Onset in Alzheimer's Disease." *The Lancet, 348* (1996):429–432.

Terri, L., and Gallagher-Thompson, D. "Cognitive-Behavioral Interventions for Treatment of Depression in Alzheimer's Patients." *Gerontologist, 31* (1991): 413–416.

Teusink, J.P., and Mahler, S. "Helping Families Cope with Alzheimer's Disease." *Hospital and Community Psychiatry, 35* (1984):152–156.

Thal, L., and Fuld, P. "Memory Enhancement with Oral Physostigmine in Alzheimer's Disease." *N. Engl. J. Med., 308* (1983):720.

Thienhaus, O.J. et al. "Biologic Markers in Alzheimer's Disease." *JAGS, 33*, no. 10 (1985):715–726.

U.S. Department of Health and Human Services. *Alzheimer's Disease: A Scientific Guide for Health Practitioners.* Publication no. 81-2251, 1980.

Volicer, L. et al. "Serotoninergic System in Dementia of the Alzheimer Type." *Arch. Neurol., 42* (Dec. 85):1158–1161.

Weiner, M. "Introduction." In *The Dementias: Diagnosis, Management, and Research* (2nd Edition), edited by Weiner, M., xix–xxiii. Washington, D.C.: American Psychiatric Press, 1996.

Weiner, M., and Gray, K. "Differential Diagnosis." In *The Dementias: Diagnosis, Management, and Research* (2nd Edition), edited by Weiner, M., 110–138. Washington, D.C.: American Psychiatric Press, 1996.

Weintraub, S. et al. "Lecithin in the Treatment of Alzheimer's Disease." *Arch. Neurol., 40* (Aug. 1983):525–528.

White, L. et al. "Prevalence of Dementia in Older Japanese-American Men in Hawaii: The Honolulu-Asia Aging Study." *JAMA, 276* (1996):955–960.

Winblad, B. et al. "Biogenic Amines in Brains of Patients with Alzheimer's Disease." In *Alzheimer's Disease: A Report of Progress in Research (Aging,* Vol. 19), edited by Corkin, S. et al., 25–34. New York: Raven Press, 1982.

Wisniewski, H.M. "Possible Viral Etiology of Neurofibrillary Changes and Neuritic Plaques." In *Alzheimer's Disease: Senile Dementia and Related Disorders (Aging,* Vol. 7), edited by Katzman, R. et al., 555–558. New York: Raven Press, 1978.

Wisniewski, H.M. "Neuritic (Senile) and Amyloid Plaques." In *Alzheimer's Disease: The Standard Reference,* edited by Reisberg, B., 57–61. New York: The Free Press, 1983.

Worden, J. William. *Grief Counseling and Grief Therapy: A Handbook for the Mental Health Practitioner.* New York: Springer, 1991.

Yates, C.M. "Aluminum and Alzheimer's Disease." In *Alzheimer's Disease: Early Recognition of Potentially Reversible Deficits,* edited by Glen A.I.M., and Whalley, L.J., 53–56. London and New York: Churchill Livingstone, 1979.

INDEX